THE
MENTAL STATUS
EXAMINATION
IN NEUROLOGY

The Mental Status Examination in Neurology

Richard L. Strub, MD
Assistant Professor of Neurology
Louisiana State University

F. William Black, PhD
Assistant Professor of Neurology
Louisiana State University

Foreword by Norman Geschwind

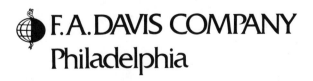
F. A. DAVIS COMPANY
Philadelphia

Library of Congress Cataloging in Publication Data

Strub, Richard L
    Mental status examination in neurology.

    Includes bibliographical references and index.
    1. Brain damage—Diagnosis. 2. Neurologic examination. 3. Psychodiagnostics. I. Black, F. William, joint author. II. Title. [DNLM: 1. Neurologic examination. 2. Nervous system diseases—Diagnosis. WL141 S925m]
RC386.2.S77   616.8'5884   76-30734
ISBN 0-8036-8208-5

Foreword

The testing of mental status has a curious, not to say anomalous, position in the examination of patients. Every medical student has had the experience of being given a long and detailed outline, or an even longer booklet, containing a seemingly endless list of items. Even if he should go to the trouble of memorizing these miniature compendia, he is likely to discover that his teachers, both neurologic and psychiatric, are disinclined to be concerned with the detailed examination, and often rely, at best, on fragments. The examinations themselves seem to differ from those in other fields of medicine. The student rapidly comes to appreciate the direct relevance of rectal tenderness to the diagnosis of appendicitis or of pulsus parodoxus to pericardial effusion. The mental examination seems to him to be much more indirectly and diffusely related to diagnostic categories.

Equally striking, or even more so, is the usual lack of direct correlation between the test items and disorders of structure or physiology. Orthopnea, swollen neck veins, rales at the lung bases, cardiac enlargement, characteristic murmurs, and auricular fibrillation not only mean congestive failure, but all the findings on examination come to blend almost imperceptibly and effortlessly with knowledge of normal cardiac structures and physiology and awareness of lawful derangements in disease. This easy understanding of the relationship of abnormal findings on examination to anatomy and physiology seems to be lacking in the mental examination.

There is, however, no reason that this situation should persist. The growth of knowledge concerning disorders of the higher functions has been rapid over the past quarter century. Not only has our ability to specify anatomic systems involved in different behaviors increased, but, even more important, we have come to a deeper understanding of the mechanisms underlying disordered function.

This book therefore represents a valuable synthesis. For the attentive reader it will yield important advantages. Not only does it shift the emphasis to those methods of examination that have proven their worth in the clinic, but it provides wherever possible a link to known anatomic and physiologic mechanisms.

Several final comments are appropriate. There is a widespread, usually tacit but often openly expressed, view that mental examination is a long and arduous task. Most physicians have learned that although a "complete" survey of the heart, lungs, abdomen and other structures can take hours, intimate knowledge of the examination and repeated practice enable them to obtain essential information in a very brief time. Those who have learned the mental examination and have practiced it often can equally well obtain vital information rapidly and efficiently when necessary. There is another common view that mental examination can be handed over to others. We should remember, however, that the real measure of a physician's usefulness lies in his capacity to make critical decisions when he is alone with the patient in the small hours of the night. Furthermore, unless he can screen patients effectively he will fail to refer intelligently to others. Finally, if the ultimate decisions lie in his hands he will fail to use adequately the opinions of his consultants unless he has a basic understanding of all aspects of his patient's problems. The newer knowledge of mental examination set forth within this book is essential, not merely to the neurologist or psychiatrist, but to all physicians.

Norman Geschwind, M.D.
James Jackson Putnam Professor of Neurology
Harvard Medical School

Preface

The primary purpose of this book is to familiarize the reader with the systematic and comprehensive mental status examination. Detailed information is provided concerning how to carry out and interpret each aspect of the exam and, where appropriate, common pitfalls in testing and interpretation are pointed out. With an understanding of the philosophy and content of this book and a period of clinical experience, the examiner will be able to administer either a brief (15 minutes) but systematic examination of the essential aspects of mental status, or carry out a more detailed comprehensive evaluation of all relevant behavioral factors. The second major purpose of the book is to help the clinician use the mental status exam data to identify patients with organic brain disease and in many instances to make specific clinical and neuroanatomic diagnoses during the initial evaluation. With these data, a more specific and oftentimes efficient neurodiagnostic workup may be arranged. A third objective is to teach the examiner to accurately describe and communicate not only the patient's cognitive and emotional deficits, but also his residual strengths. By this summarization of the patient's current functioning, it is possible for the clinician more appropriately to manage the patient and to help the patient and his family plan for his social and vocational readjustment.

Richard L. Strub
F. William Black

Contents

CHAPTER 1

The Mental Status Examination: A Rationale and Overview

Human behavior is an extremely complex multifaceted entity. The understanding of its disruption in brain disease has proved to be a substantial and oftentimes frustrating problem to the clinician who is faced with the tasks of diagnosis and management. The patients with organically related changes in intellectual or emotional behavior unfortunately have often fallen just outside the limits of both psychiatry and neurology. Behavioral problems within this somewhat uncharted borderland have long been subsumed under the rubric of "the organic brain syndromes," a vague and overly inclusive term covering any possible behavior change from brain damage or dysfunction. The term has little clinical utility for specific diagnosis, description, or patient management. In recent years, however, there has been a renewed interest in these organic mental syndromes and it is now possible to understand many of these conditions and to assign specific patterns of behavioral deficits to specific diseases or to damage in particular regions of the brain.

Although the study of the neurobehavioral disorders has not yet reached the stage of fashionable medical popularity of arteriosclerotic heart disease, cancer, or immunologic disorders of infancy, the magnitude and social impact of these disorders must not be underestimated. The neuropsychiatric or neurobehavioral syndromes are very common in both hospital and office practice. Dementia, aphasia, confusional states, and learning disabilities are not rare conditions that each medical student dutifully learns about in medical school and then fruitlessly searches for in clinical practice for the rest of his career. Quite the opposite is true, these are problems that the average clinician sees every day, but has typically never learned about in school. Hopefully, tomorrow's students will recognize early dementia as readily as they do pheochromocytomas or pseudohypoparathyroidism. Primary neurologic diseases account for at least 30 percent of all first admissions to psychiatric hospitals,[2] while intellectual deterioration (dementia) has been reported to be the third most frequent cause for hospital admission among all patients with suspected neurologic disease.[1]

For the examiner to adequately understand organically based behavior change and to allow the application of this understanding to individual clinical cases, he must utilize a systematic behavioral examination. This evaluation is the mental status examination. It is an orderly assessment of the important cognitive and emotional functions that are commonly and characteristically disturbed in patients with organic brain disease.

Because the mental status examination is a component of the comprehensive neurologic evaluation, it is important that the clinician be able to determine when inclusion of the mental status exam is appropriate. ·Just as the patient with otitis externa does not routinely require an electrocardiogram, the patient with a peripheral neuropathy does not usually need a full mental status examination. Conversely, the patient vomiting blood requires an immediate upper GI series, just as the patient complaining of memory difficulty needs a comprehensive mental status exam. There are many patients in whom full mental status testing is definitely indicated. Patients with documented brain lesions such as tumors, trauma, vascular accident, and so forth minimally should have a screening mental status evaluation to document any cognitive or emotional changes. It is a sad but true commentary on the current state of neurobehavioral knowledge in medicine that subtle (and sometimes gross) deficits secondary to known brain lesions are overlooked or considered inconsequential by the primary physician. Many patients with mild aphasias or memory deficits after craniotomy, increased irritability and decreased ability to concentrate after head trauma, or marked emotional lability following infectious neurologic disease are released from the hospital without recognition of these cognitive and emotional deficits. Such patients frequently become emotionally frustrated, have difficulty with social readjustment, and are unable to carry out the demands of home and vocation. An early eduction of the neurobehavioral sequelae of the known neurologic disorder helps to explain the totality of the patient's disability to family and employers, thus preventing needless frustration on the patient's part. Such documentation is of immeasurable aid in planning social and vocational rehabilitation when indicated.

There is another large group of patients in which mental testing is indicated. These are patients in whom a brain lesion is suspected because of recent onset of seizures, headaches, behavior change, or head trauma. Brain tumors, subdural hematomas, small infarcts, or cerebral atrophy may be undetected on the routine neurologic examination because of their location or discrete nature during early stages, whereas the cognitive effects of these lesions may often be readily apparent on a complete mental status examination. Thus, the inclusion of the mental status examination

2

as a component of the initial neurologic evaluation may significantly increase the probability of detecting neurologic disease when present and effectively ruling it out when absent. We recently saw a 46-year-old man who was admitted to the infectious disease isolation unit because of fever, "jumbled" speech, and "confusion." His admitting diagnosis was "probable encephalitis." Subsequent mental status testing the morning following admission revealed an aphasia rather than a confusional state. As the finding of aphasia is almost pathognomonic of significant left hemisphere disease, a left carotid arteriogram was performed and a large subdural hematoma was found. With appropriate treatment (surgery), the patient had an uneventful and complete recovery. Had the correct diagnosis not been made quickly, the patient could well have died without appropriate treatment and with the incorrect diagnosis of "devastating herpes simplex encephalitis."

In patients in whom the diagnosis of neurologic disease is difficult or equivocal, the mental status examination may be as specific in documenting a brain lesion and indicating its location as the elicitation of a Babinski reflex. Accordingly, it is essential that these patients receive a comprehensive mental status examination as a part of the complete neurodiagnostic workup.

We feel that a full mental status examination should be carried out on all psychiatric patients, particularly those whose psychiatric symptoms appear rather acutely and are superimposed upon a life history of normal emotional functioning. Organic brain disease frequently presents initially as emotional and behavioral change and thereby comes first to the attention of the psychiatrist or to the family physician in the guise of psychiatric symptomology. This presentation is especially characteristic of frontal and temporal tumors, hydrocephalus, or cortical atrophy. The most common behavioral symptom seen in these patients is depression. Brain disease should be strongly suspected in any patient with a middle or late life depression which is not clearly reactive in nature. In our clinical practice we have seen a large number of patients being treated with psychotrophic drugs, psychotherapy, electroshock, and long term psychiatric hospitalization for an apparent depressive illness who have, in fact, demonstrated clear signs of primary organic disease on mental status testing and subsequent neurodiagnostic procedures (C.A.T. scan). Although some organic patients will develop a reactive depression with their primary illness and will show an initial positive response to such therapeutic measures, it is far more economical, efficacious, and appropriate to spend 15 minutes during the initial interview doing a complete mental status examination than to embark upon a lengthy, expensive, and sometimes inappropriate treatment regimen.

The differentiation between psychiatric and organic disease is not always possible and is oftentimes difficult. The functionally depressed patient with psychomotor retardation may perform poorly on some aspects of the mental status examination and in this way present the picture of a pseudo-dementia. Other patients have elements of both organic and functional disease and at times it requires considerable effort to separate the respective components even on careful examination. The mental status examination is not infallible even in the hands of an experienced examiner. The fact remains, however, that the majority of these patients with borderland problems will be correctly classified if appropriate mental testing is done.

A final group of patients in whom mental status screening is extremely important is those who initially present or are presented by their family with vague behavioral complaints which are difficult to clinically substantiate and quantify. Complaints such as memory problems, difficulties in concentration, declining interest in family or work, or various physical complaints without organic etiology all should alert the clinician to the possibility of organic brain disease. The determination of the etiology of such problems involves a difficult differentiation among functional, neurologic, or other medical etiologies. However, it can often be readily made with the aid of data provided by the mental status examination.

The clinician must appreciate that the mental status examination must be arranged in a systematic and hierarchical fashion. In this sense the mental status examination is analogous to any comprehensive medical examination. When the patient shows impaired performance on early sections of the examination, for example in language, it will be difficult, if not impossible, for the examiner to accurately assess verbal memory (an extremely important function) or any other function requiring language. The language disturbance (aphasia) interferes with the patient's ability to comprehend and respond to items used in this testing. Similarly, the patient who is organically inattentive will miss important details during much of the higher level testing, especially the memory and calculation items. If the mental status examination is carried out in a haphazard manner without regard for the hierarchical nature of cognitive performance, erroneous conclusions will be drawn. The exam must be performed in an orderly way with the assessment of basic processes such as the level of consciousness, attention, and vigilance first and the higher level functions such as abstract reasoning and special cognitive functions tested last.

The mental status examination as presented in this book may seem exceptionally detailed and it may appear that the exam would take hours to complete in its entirety. This conception is similar to the beginning clinician's first attempts to understand the evaluation of the cranial nerves or the brachial plexus. When first learning to administer the exam, it is wise to evaluate several patients fully to gain experience in carrying out and interpreting all test items. With time, the examination can be completed rapidly (15 to 20 minutes) and will yield much valuable data. In Appendix 2, we have summarized the examination and indicated how the exam can

4

be tailored to meet the demands of the situation and the particular patient.

In many cases a brief exam will provide definitive data to allow the correct diagnosis and appropriate and often life saving medical treatment. As an example of the ease in administering a meaningful examination in a brief period of time, a psychiatrist, recently called in the middle of the night to see a patient who was "talking out of his head," started to examine the patient's language and found that the patient was actually aphasic and not psychotic. At this point the psychiatrist consulted the neurologist and had the patient admitted to a service other than the psychiatric unit. In this case the psychiatrist had properly evaluated the patient and averted an inappropriate type of hospitalization and treatment, and possibly saved the patient's life. We recently were called to see a similar case in which a young man had been admitted to the psychiatric service because he was answering questions inappropriately and did not make sense in conversation. This behavior had initially disturbed his parents who had brought him to the emergency room. Upon evaluation, the patient had little, if any, comprehension of language and was producing fluent paraphasic speech (aphasia). Neurodiagnostic evaluation revealed a large hematoma in the dominant temporal lobe. His "craziness" was due to a readily apparent organic disorder and his psychiatric hospitalization had resulted from the admitting physician's lack of recognition of the patient's condition. In this case, demonstration of a typical pattern of aphasia indicated not only the diagnosis of organic disease but strongly suggested the location of the lesion.

These clinical examples illustrate that even a brief exam in the hands of the skilled examiner may be of critical clinical importance. In other patients, however, a more comprehensive assessment will be required. The patient referred after a head injury required a detailed elucidation of cognitive strengths and deficits to allow for appropriate social and vocational rehabilitation. The need for a comprehensive mental status examination is amply demonstrated in the following case. The physical medicine service requested consultation on a 32-year-old female who had suffered a severe basilar skull facture several months previously and was not progressing satisfactorily in the inpatient rehabilitation program. There were also questions of "difficult" and "uncooperative" behavior. Mental status testing revealed an apathetic patient without insight or concern who had moderately impaired attention and vigilance. Multiple significant cognitive deficits were demonstrated including a mild general dementia, moderately impaired recent and remote memory, severely impaired new learning ability, and a moderate to severe impairment of all higher level cognitive functions (abstraction, calculations, and so forth). The documentation of an organic behavior change and significant cognitive deficits helped to explain both the patient's difficult ward behavior and her inability to fully participate in a demanding rehabilitation program. Her rehabilitation program had to be restructured and her goals altered because of the appreciation of the extent of her cognitive and behavioral deficits.

In complicated situations when extensive and quantitative data regarding cognitive and emotional functioning are required for proper patient management, consultation should be obtained from relevant ancillary professionals. These include psychologists and speech pathologists. The bedside or office mental status examination as outlined in this book is very effective in diagnosing organic disease and in evaluating major areas of deficit. By its nature the examination is qualitative and does not offer the advantages of standardized quantitative data which are necessary for evaluating subtle deficits, planning for comprehensive rehabilitation efforts, and assessing improvements in performance. The neuropsychologist can provide this data and additional valuable consultation when a definitive evaluation is required for whatever reason. In patients with significant communication problems, referral to the speech pathologist for comprehensive evaluation of language, possible treatment, and family counseling to facilitate communication between the patient and other family members is important. Chapter 11 deals in detail with the specifics of the consultation process. Every clinician should be aware of the availability and scope of such ancillary services and utilize them when appropriate for the benefit of the patient.

REFERENCES

1. Harner, R. N.: EEG evaluation of the patient with dementia, in Benson, D. F., and Blumer, D. (eds.): Psychiatric Aspects of Neurologic Disease. Grune and Stratton, New York, 1975, pp. 63–82.
2. Malzberg, B.: Important statistical data about mental illness, in Arieti, S. (ed.): American Handbook of Psychiatry, Vol. 1. Basic Books, New York, 1959, pp. 161–174.

CHAPTER 2

Levels of Consciousness

The initial step in a mental status examination is the determination of the patient's level of consciousness. This basic brain function determines the patient's ability to relate, both to himself and to his environment. Any disturbance of this elementary function will almost invariably affect the higher level mental processes that constitute the major portion of the examination. The term consciousness is multifaceted and in testing it is important to make a distinction between the content of consciousness and basic arousal.[6] Content refers to higher cortical functioning, whereas arousal refers to the activation of the cortex from the brain stem reticular formation and the diffuse thalamic projection system. The aspects of content and arousal can vary independently and the final level of consciousness represents a dynamic balance of cortical and the ascending activating systems. This chapter deals with the clinical aspects of basic arousal, whereas discussion of changes in the content of consciousness is included in subsequent sections of the book.

TERMINOLOGY AND EVALUATION

There are many general terms used to describe the basic levels or states of consciousness. These levels represent points on a continuum from full alertness to deep coma. Most clinicians distinguish four principal levels: (1) alertness, (2) lethargy or somnolence, (3) stupor or semicoma, and (4) coma. Alertness implies that the patient is awake and fully aware of normal external and internal stimuli. Barring paralysis the patient can respond normally to such stimuli. The alert patient is able to interact in a meaningful way with the examiner. In cases of total paralysis, eye contact or eye movement may be adequate to establish this interaction. Because there are unusual coma-like states in which alertness is simulated, we feel that an observation of alertness should be predicated upon the clinician's impression that meaningful interpersonal interaction is taking place. Alertness, per se, is a quite different aspect of conscious behavior from the capacity to focus attention, a topic to be discussed in detail in Chapter 3.

Lethargy is a state in which the patient is not fully alert and tends to drift off to sleep when not specifically stimulated. In such patients, spontaneous movements are decreased and awareness is limited. When aroused, these patients usually do not pay close attention to the examiner. The lethargic patient often loses the train of thought and wanders from topic to topic in conversation. It is difficult to assess memory, calculations, and abstract thinking in these patients because of their inattention and wandering thought processes. If a full mental status examination is carried out in a lethargic patient, the results must be interpreted with some caution.

The terms stupor and semicoma are used to describe patients who respond only to rather persistent and vigorous stimulation. The stuporous patient does not rouse spontaneously and when aroused by the examiner is able only to groan and move restlessly in the bed. In such a patient there is extensive brain dysfunction and thus no meaningful assessment of the content of mental functioning is possible. Coma is a term traditionally reserved for those patients who are completely unarousable. In coma, the patient will neither respond to any external stimulation nor respond spontaneously to an internal stimulus. If coma is thus defined as a state in which no evidence of behavioral response to stimulation is present, the term can serve as an absolute end point on the scale of consciousness or arousability. These latter two states will not be further discussed here; the interested reader is referred to Plum and Posner (1972)[6] and Fisher (1969)[2] for extensive discussions of stupor and coma.

Each of the above mentioned terms is qualitative in nature and each general term encompasses a wide range of possible points on the continuum of consciousness. Such terms lack the objectivity and reliability that can be achieved with a more complete assessment scheme. We suggest amending any qualitative term such as "lethargy" with a series of short statements that describe the patient's actual behavioral response. First, indicate the intensity of stimulation needed to arouse the patient: (1) calling the patient's name in a normal conversational tone, (2) calling in a loud voice, (3) light touch on the arm, (4) vigorous shaking of the patient's shoulder, and (5) painful stimulation. Second, describe the patient's response: (1) degree and quality of movement, (2) content and coherence of speech, and (3) presence of eye opening and eye contact with the examiner. Finally, describe what the patient does upon cessation of stimulation.

This information can be recorded in a single statement, for example, (1) patient lethargic: name called in a normal tone of voice, patient opened eyes, pulled self part way up in bed, mumbled "Why ya bothering me," then closed eyes and went back to sleep. (2) Patient very lethargic: Responds to loud shouting with restless movements of all extremities and brief eye opening. Speech is mumbled and incoherent. When stimulation discontinued, patient returns to sleep. (3) Patient stuporous: Does not respond to voice, but will respond to vigorous shaking of shoulder accompanied by loud calling of patient's name. Patient responds with a groan and aimless movement of left extremities. Eyes remain closed.

This type of description provides much more data on the patient's arousability and capacity for interaction than a simple term like "lethargy" or "stupor." It is helpful to make a chart in the progress notes so that a rapid assessment of changing level of consciousness can be made. Table 2-1 is an example of such a chart made about a patient with head trauma who had a subdural hematoma. As nurse and doctor shifts change, subtle changes in the patient's condition are easily appreciated by comparing the notes of previous observers. The practicality of this reporting system has been recently demonstrated in patients with head trauma where level of consciousness must be assessed at frequent intervals.[8] This system is applicable to any patient whose illness causes a decrease in the level of awareness.

ANATOMY AND CLINICAL IMPLICATIONS

The basic brain structure responsible for arousal is the ascending activating system. This system originates in the brain stem reticular formation and extends to the cortex via the diffuse or nonspecific thalamic projection system.[5]

There is a group of specialized reticular neurons in the tegmental portion of the midbrain and upper pons that has the specific capacity to activate higher centers. These cells are located in a perimedian portion in the brain stem and receive collateral input from most ascending and decending fiber systems. Stimulation to the skin of the hand, for example, will send information to the activating system as well as the normal sensory nuclei in the thalamus. This reticular stimulation alerts widespread areas of cortex and subcortex to the fact that an external stimulus is being applied. By this mechanism the activating system maintains a constant, albeit fluctuating stimulation of the higher centers, particularly the cortex. Without this steady input the cortex cannot function efficiently and thus the patient cannot think clearly, learn effectively, or relate meaningfully. Any damage or suppression of this system renders the patient difficult to arouse and inefficient in his performance. Specific lesions such as infarcts or hemorrhages of the reticular formation lead to total disruption of arousal and, thus, coma.

TABLE 2-1. Patient's responses to stimulation

	Level of consciousness	Stimulus necessary to rouse patient	Movement	Vocalization	Eye opening	Comments
8:00 p.m.	Lethargy	Loud voice	Moved all limbs Got up on elbow	Mumbled something about being tired	Yes, with eye contact	Odor of alcohol on breath
12:00 a.m.	Lethargy	Loud voice plus gentle shaking	Moved all limbs No attempt to rise	Incoherent mumbling	Yes, but no sustained eye contact	Questionable Babinski sign
4:00 a.m.	Stupor	Loud voice plus vigorous shaking	Slight movement of all extremities, but right arm not moving well	Groans	Attempted to open eyes to command	Left pupil larger than right, not as reactive. Now positive Babinski on right

10

Pressure on the midbrain from hippocampal or uncal herniation will cause a change in the level of consciousness which starts as lethargy but may progress to coma. Drug intoxication, disturbances in metabolic balance, or sepsis cause alterations in both reticular and cortical functioning. This leads to alterations not only in arousal, but also in the content of consciousness. If there is damage to the extension of the brain stem reticular system in the thalamus or hypothalamus, the full picture of coma will not result. Such lesions disconnect the reticulocortical pathways and cause the patients to display various interesting alterations in arousal that simulate awareness. Since the brain stem portion of the system is intact, reticular activity innervates the nuclei of the extraocular nerves and the patients can open their eyes and look about. They are not, however, able to sufficiently stimulate the cortex to produce voluntary movement or speech. These patients are in a coma-like state which must be fully appreciated before attempting to make further assessment.

This group of unusual coma-like states is interesting because of the nature and degree of disturbed awareness. Some authors combine all such cases under the rubrics of akinetic mutism or persistent vegetative states, while other writers prefer to separate the patients into many subcategories. Regardless of the terminology employed, the pathology and clinical appearance of each subcategory is relatively distinct and can usually be recognized by a thorough examiner. The primary feature of these disorders is the patient's uncanny appearance of awareness. The patients lie in bed with their eyes open and look about the room. Eye contact with others is variable. Sometimes eye movements seem random, but on other occasions real interpersonal eye contact appears to take place. Other than this somewhat unnerving visual scanning, the patients remain relatively immobile and mute. It is the dichotomy between this apparent visual alertness and the lack of speech and movement that differentiates this group of patients from those in stupor or coma.

Regardless of their superficial similarity, each subgroup has its own distinct features and it is often possible to clinically differentiate the various states. The term akinetic mutism seems best reserved for cases in which damage is restricted to either the midbrain subthalamic region or to the septal region. The midbrain lesion causes a syndrome which is described as an apathetic akinetic mutism. These patients are difficult to arouse, but once aroused can move all extremities, mutter a few intelligible words, and look directly at the examiner for a few moments. They then turn away or drift back into sleep. Subtle muscle stretch reflex changes, possible extensor toe signs, extraocular muscle involvement, and pupillary abnormalities may be seen. This condition was originally described in a patient with a third ventricular cyst,[1] but the most common cause is occlusion of the small vessels entering the brain stem from the tip of the basilar artery.[7] This lesion interrupts the ascending activating system, but not the corticospinal and corticobulbar tracts. Accordingly the patient is able to open his eyes and make some movement and sound, but not to respond fully.

Patients with lesions involving the septal area, anterior hypothalamus, cingulate gyri, or bilateral orbital frontal cortex are also akinetic and mute, but appear much more alert. They are awake most of the time, and their eyes remain open when awake. These patients often have violent outbursts during arousal, but this is not seen in all cases. Coma vigil is a term that has been used to describe such patients. This syndrome is seen with rupture of anterior communicating artery aneurysms, deep frontal lobe tumors, and anterior cingulate gyrus tumors. These patients may have increased reflexes in the legs with Babinski signs from corticospinal tract involvement, difficulty with temperature control from anterior hypothalamic damage, and primitive reflexes (snout and grasp) from mesial frontal lobe damage. They do not have pupillary or extraocular muscle paresis. These neurologic signs plus the more apparent alertness of these patients will frequently differentiate them clinically from the apathetic akinetic mute patients.

Patients with diffuse damage to the cortical mantle from anoxia, hypoglycemia, or from circulatory or metabolic embarrassment will frequently survive in a state clinically similar to coma vigil. Their eyes are open and randomly survey the room. Brain stem reflexes are intact, but there is bilateral decortication with double hemiplegia and primitive reflexes. This condition has been termed the apallic state[4] because of the diffuse damage to the neocortex or neopallium. Because of the dramatic neurologic deficit, this state should be easily distinguished from the akinetic mute states.

The term persistent vegetative state has recently been used to describe patients surviving severe head injury who remain clinically similar to the apallic patients.[3] The brain lesions are widespread at both the cortical and subcortical levels and neurologic findings differ in each case dependent upon the specific loci of lesions.

The locked-in syndrome[6] must also be recognized and differentiated from the above states. In this condition there is a lesion (hemorrhage or infarct) in the upper pontine tegmentum that interrupts all corticospinal and corticobulbar fibers at the level of the abducens and facial nuclei. Clinically, the patient is unable to speak, swallow, smile, or move his limbs. In some cases, lateral gaze is also paralyzed. The entire central nervous system above the level of the lesion is intact and the patient is literally disconnected from his motor system. He is "locked-in" and is able to communicate with his onlookers only by eye movements.

Table 2-2 is a composite of the clinical features of each of these coma-

TABLE 2-2. Diagnostic features of coma-like states

Diagnosis	Level of consciousness	Voluntary movement	Speech	Eye responses	Limb tone	Reflexes
Akinetic mute (apathetic—midbrain)	Lethargy	Little and infrequent but when sufficiently stimulated can move *all* extremities purposefully.	With stimulation can produce normal, short phrases.	Open when stimulated. Usually good eye contact	Usually normal, sometimes slight increase.	Can be normal. Occasionally asymmetrical with pathologic reflexes.
Akinetic mute (coma—vigil—septal)	Wakeful with occasional outbursts. Some patients are somnolent.	Little but purposeful, arms usually move much better than legs.	Little, can occasionally produce normal phrases. Also can have outbursts of unintelligible utterances.	Open during much of the day in most patients. Eye contact variable.	Often increased in legs.	Frequently have increased leg reflexes. Babinski signs, snout, grasp often present.
Apallic state (decorticate)	Awake, no meaningful interaction with environment.	No or little purposeful movement, mostly reflex or mass movements.	None or occasional grunting.	Open, searching but no real eye contact.	Increased in all extremities. Extremities often in flexion.	Increased in all extremities with pathologic reflexes.
Persistent vegetative state	Awake, no or little interaction with the environment.	Usually little or none, depending upon areas of brain damaged. Mostly primitive postural reflexes.	None or occasional grunts or groans. Some patients produce a few words.	Open, searching but no real eye contact.	Variable, usually increased. Extremities often in flexion.	Variable, usually increased with pathologic reflexes.
Locked-in syndrome	Awake and alert, able to communicate meaningfully with examiners by eye movement.	None or slight except for eye movement.	None	Open with normal following and good eye contact. Some patients have restricted lateral gaze.	Increased	Increased in all extremities.

13

like states. These features plus the clinical history should enable the examiner to differentiate most of these complicated cases.

A final condition which deserves mention in this section is the state of psychogenic unresponsiveness (hysteric coma-like state). This condition constitutes 1 percent of all patients presenting to a medical emergency room in a comatose state.[6] Careful examination reveals normal respiration, heart rate, and blood pressure. Muscle tone is usually decreased, but there is frequently an inconsistent limb tone. All bulbar reflexes (Doll's phenomenon, caloric stimulation, gag, corneal, and pupil) are intact. Muscle stretch reflexes are symmetrical and no pathologic reflexes are present. A normal medical and neurologic examination strongly suggests that the condition is psychogenic. Frequently the patient will make inconsistent responses such as blinking on corneal testing before the cornea is touched. Any inconsistent response gives the examiner additional confidence that he is not dealing with an organic coma. Do not diagnose psychogenic unresponsiveness too hastily; the misdiagnosis of a true coma as hysteria is far more serious than the reverse.

All the conditions discussed above represent disturbances of arousal that are caused by brain lesions or psychiatric illness. Not all alterations in levels of alertness are pathologic, however. Sleep, for instance, is a natural fluctuation in the level of consciousness. Any degree of fatigue or sleepiness can adversely effect performance on mental status testing even though an organic lesion is not present. Patients with brain disease will continue to have an underlying diurnal sleep/wake cycle which is superimposed upon any organic decrease in alertness. It may be difficult to determine the relative effects of sleep and pathologic alterations in the level of consciousness, but the examiner must consider both of these factors in his evaluation. For example, the head trauma patient who is difficult to arouse on morning rounds may only be asleep and not suffering from increasing intracranial pressure. In these critical cases, observed level of awareness is not the only clinical factor determining the necessity of therapeutic intervention. The patient's neurologic status and overall hospital course must also be considered.

SUMMARY

Consciousness is the most rudimentary of all mental functions, and its level must be determined first in any mental status examination. Any alteration in the level of consciousness will decrease efficiency of cortical functioning, and thereby significantly decrease the validity of the subsequent steps in the mental status examination. In the patient with diminished alertness, only the more obvious changes in higher cognitive function can be documented.

The arousal aspect of consciousness is controlled by the ascending activating system. Any damage or dysfunction of this subcortical system alters alertness and thus, secondarily, affects cortical activity.

REFERENCES

1. Cairns, H., Oldfield, R., Pennybacker, J., and Whitteridge, D.: Akinetic mutism with an epidermoid cyst of the third ventricle. Brain 64:273, 1941.
2. Fisher, G.: The neurological examination of the comatose patient. Acta Neurol. Scand. (Suppl.) 36:1, 1969.
3. Jennett, B., and Plum, F.: Persistent vegetative state after brain damage. Lancet 1:734, 1972.
4. Kretschmer, E.: Das appalische syndrom. Z. Gesamte Neurol. Psychiat. 189: 576, 1940.
5. Magoun, H.: The Waking Brain. Charles C Thomas, Springfield, Ill., 1963.
6. Plum, F., and Posner, J.: Diagnosis of Stupor and Coma. F. A. Davis, Philadelphia, 1972.
7. Segarra, J., and Angelo, J.: Anatomical determinants of behavior change, in Benton, A. (ed.): Behavioral Change in Cerebral Vascular Disease. Harper and Row, New York, 1970, pp. 3-14.
8. Teasdale, G., and Jennett, B.: Assessment of coma and impaired consciousness. Lancet 2:81, 1974.

CHAPTER 3

Attention

After a determination of the level of consciousness, a careful assessment of attention is the next step of the formal mental status examination. The patient's ability to sustain attention over time must be established before the more complex functions such as memory, language, and abstract thinking are evaluated. It is of no value to ask the patient to remember the details of a story if he is repeatedly distracted by the nurse passing in the hall, a noise in the next room, or cars in the street. When a patient is inattentive and distractable, he is unable to assimilate the information to be tested.

Attention refers to the patient's ability to attend to a specific stimulus without being distracted by extraneous environmental stimuli. This capacity for focusing on a single stimulus is in contrast to the concept of alertness. Alertness is a more basic arousal process in which the awake patient is able to respond to any stimulus in the environment. The alert, but inattentive patient will be attracted to any novel sound, movement, or event occurring in his vicinity; while the attentive patient is able to screen out irrelevant stimuli. Attention presupposes alertness, but alertness does not necessarily imply attentiveness.

Vigilance (concentration) is a term that refers to the ability to sustain attention over an extended period of time. For the purpose of mental status testing, a vigilant period of 30 seconds is all that is typically required. This capacity to concentrate is very important in carrying out intellectual endeavors and may be impaired in organic as well as emotional disorders. There are, however, certain situations and jobs which require unusually long periods of sustained attention (e.g., airport radar operators or inspectors on an assembly line). Information concerning this aspect of vigilance must be ascertained from the patient's history, for it is not practical to test on routine examination.

The concept of inattention (distractability) is applied to two distinct clinical situations. The first refers to the patient who is clinically inattentive or is unable to sustain sufficient attention to succeed on the simple tests of attention discussed below. The second type of inattention is a specific inattention to stimuli on the side of the body opposite a unilateral brain lesion. This inattention can be extreme to the point that the patient becomes unaware of people approaching on his inattentive side or fails to dress or shave on that side. This marked inattention is called unilateral neglect and is one aspect of organic denial. Inattention of this marked degree is less common than a more subtle form where the patient is only inattentive to stimuli on one side during bilateral simultaneous stimulation. For instance, the patient would acknowledge a touch on one arm alone (the arm opposite the intact hemisphere) even though the examiner had touched both arms with equal intensity.

EVALUATION

Observation

Alertness has been previously evaluated during that portion of the mental status examination concerning levels of consciousness (Chap. 2). Considerable information regarding the patient's general attentiveness may be obtained by merely observing his behavior and noting any evidence of distractability or difficulty in attending to the examiner.

History

A patient who is having difficulty concentrating on his work or other routine tasks is usually able to tell the examiner about his problem. A simple inquiry as to his ability to concentrate or sustain attention may provide revealing data.

Digit Repetition

The patient's basic level of attention can be readily assessed utilizing the digit repetition test. Adequate performance on this task ensures that the patient is able to attend to a verbal stimulus and to sustain attention for the period of time required to repeat the digits.

Directions. Tell the patient, "I am going to say some simple numbers. Listen carefully and when I am finished, say the same numbers after me." Present the digits in a normal tone of voice at a rate of one digit per second. Take care not to group digits either in pairs (e.g., 2-6, 5-9) or in sequences which could serve as an aid to repetition (e.g., in the telephone number form, 376-8439). Numbers should be presented randomly without natural sequences (e.g., not 2-4-6-8). Begin with a two number sequence and continue until the patient fails.

Test Items.

3-7
7-4-9
8-5-2-1
2-9-6-8-3
5-7-1-9-4-6
8-1-5-9-3-6-2
3-9-8-2-5-1-4-7
7-2-8-5-4-6-7-3-9

Scoring. The typical patient of average intelligence can repeat five to seven digits without difficulty. Repetition of less than five digits by a nonretarded patient without obvious aphasia indicates defective attention.

Vigilance

A simple test of vigilance which can be readily administered at the bedside is the random letter test. This test consists of a series of random letters among which a target letter appears with greater than random frequency. The patient is required to indicate whenever the target letter is spoken by the examiner.

Directions. Tell the patient, "I am going to read you a long series of letters. Whenever you hear the letter A indicate by tapping the desk with this pencil." Read the following letter list in a normal tone at a rate of one letter per second.

Test Items.

L T P E A O A I C T D A L A A

A N I A B F S A M R Z E O A D

P A K L A U C J T O E A B A A

Z Y F M U S A H E V A A R A T

Scoring. There are no standardized levels of performance for this test. The average person should complete the task without error. Examples of common organic errors are: (1) failure to indicate when the target letter has been presented (omission error), (2) indication made when a nontarget letter has been presented (commission error), and (3) failure to stop tapping with the presentation of subsequent nontarget letters (perseveration error).

Inattention and Neglect

Unilateral inattention (suppression or extinction) should be tested in the routine sensory examination utilizing double (bilateral) simultaneous stimulation.

Directions. Double simultaneous stimulation is tested in all major sensory modalities. In tactile testing, corresponding points on both sides of the body are touched simultaneously with equal intensity. Visual testing is done by having the patient face the examiner and fix his gaze at a point on the examiner's face. The examiner then moves his fingers in both right and left peripheral fields. Auditory testing is carried out by the examiner standing behind the patient and providing a stimulus of equal intensity to each ear. Snapping the fingers which is commonly employed is not an optimal auditory stimulus as very few examiners can snap the fingers on each hand with equal intensity.

Before undertaking bilateral simultaneous stimulation, the examiner must ensure that sensation for each modality is intact bilaterally. If one side is inferior on unilateral testing, defects during simultaneous testing do not necessarily reflect inattention.

Extinction is present when the patient suppresses the stimuli from one side of the body. Extinction may occur in all modalities (polymodal neglect) or be restricted to a single modality. With tactile stimulation, there is also often a distal extinction when a single limb is stimulated simultaneously both proximally and distally.[1] When extinction is elicited, the degree of inattention can be assessed by increasing the magnitude of the stimulus on the inattentive side.

ANATOMY AND CLINICAL IMPLICATIONS

The basic anatomic structures responsible for maintaining an alert state are the brain stem reticular activating system and the diffuse thalamic projection system (the diencephalic extension of the reticular formation).[5] The arousal system is more properly called the ascending activating system because specific reticular fibers are found principally in the brain stem portion.

The mechanism by which this ascending activation is focused and extraneous stimuli are screened out is less certain. Cortical stimulation can definitely influence the activity in the ascending system, so it is probable that attention is a balance between ascending (reticulocortical) activation and cortical (corticoreticular) modulation.[5] The importance of cortical influence in focusing attention is demonstrated in the experience of every student. Concentration while studying frequently requires considerable conscious voluntary effort; this effort is cortical in origin, probably originating in the frontal lobes. The limbic system is also an integral part of the attention process; limbic input adds emotional importance to the object of attention. The child watching a cartoon and the adult watching an

X-rated movie are stimulated to attention by the pleasure and excitement generated by the spectacle. The student studying for an exam is aided in his need to concentrate by a fear of failure or a drive to succeed. These limbic influences are important and may be the critical factor that facilitates the screening out of extraneous stimuli. The principle stimulus is of greater emotional value than the incidental events in the environment and therefore attracts greater attention.

Since attention represents a complex interaction of limbic, neocortical, and ascending activating functions, damage in many areas of the brain can disrupt the ability to attend. Damage to the ascending activating system itself usually causes alterations in the level of consciousness. In such patients, alterations in attention are directly related to the more basic deficit in alertness. Inattention from lesions in the midbrain activating system is probably clinically rare, although a rather profound unilateral inattention has been experimentally produced in monkeys with lesions in the midbrain.[7] Some of the patients who survived the encephalitis epidemic of 1918–1921 associated with Von Economo's influenza were left with lesions in the reticular substance of the pons and medulla. These patients developed a behavior pattern characterized by hyperactivity and distractability which was called "organic driveness."[4] This state is clinically similar to that seen in some hyperactive children.

Probably the most common cause of decreased attention and vigilance in a hospital population is diffuse brain dysfunction. This dysfunction is usually caused by metabolic disturbance, drug intoxication, postsurgical states, and systemic infection. In these confusional states, all cells in the central nervous system are affected. Another common cause of inattention is extensive bilateral cortical damage of any etiology (e.g., atrophy, multiple infarcts, encephalitis, or head trauma). The patient with advanced cortical disease is inattentive and extremely distractable. Any new stimulus in his vicinity will quickly draw his attention; he becomes "stimulus bound" and unable to screen out irrelevant stimuli. It is in such patients that the cortical role in focusing and maintaining attention is best illustrated.

Patients with bilateral lesions of the frontal lobes or the limbic system (e.g., Korsakoff's syndrome) have a type of inattention characterized by indifference and perseveration. Clinically, they are apathetic toward their surroundings and test items per se have no particular interest to them. Such patients usually perform well on the digit repetition task, but will not accurately complete the random letter test. The patient will often omit an A at the end of a long sequence (e.g., U C J T O E A) because his attention has wandered. The frontal lobe patient also has great difficulty shifting from one pattern of response to another; this deficit results in perseveration. This perseveration is commonly seen behaviorally and on the random letter test. The series E V A A R A T may be failed in the following way (italic letters indicate patient's taps) E V *A A R A T*.

Right hemisphere lesions have a stronger effect upon attention than do left sided lesions. Denial, unilateral neglect, and extinction on double simultaneous stimulation are all more prominent with right hemisphere lesions.[3,6] The reason for this peculiar quality of the right hemisphere is not known. It is possible that reticulocortical or corticoreticular fibers are more dense in the right hemisphere, although there is no currently available pathologic evidence that this is true.

Contralateral inattention to double simultaneous stimulation is seen with parietal lesions of either hemisphere. The damage to parietal tissue apparently reduces reticulocortical interaction on the damaged side, thus allowing the intact hemisphere an advantage in the stimulus rivalry.[2]

There are many functional mood alterations that can affect attention. Anxiety causes distractability and difficulty concentrating, while depression produces disinterest and reduced arousal. All such mood changes will hinder performance on attention tasks and generally decrease attention.

SUMMARY

Attention is an interplay between brain stem and cortical activity that allows the patient to focus on a specific task to the exclusion of irrelevant stimuli. Both functional and organic illness can disrupt attention and cause a failure of vigilance. Assessment of attention must be done early in the mental status examination because the testing of many subsequent functions relies on its integrity.

REFERENCES

1. Critchley, M.: The Parietal Lobes. Edward Arnold and Company, London, 1953.
2. Denny-Brown, D., Meyers, J., and Horenstein, S.: The significance of perceptual rivalry resulting from parietal lesions. Brain 75:433, 1952.
3. Gainotti, G.: Emotional behavior and hemispheric side of lesion. Cortex 8:41, 1972.
4. Kahn, E., and Cohen, L.: Organic driveness: A brainstem syndrome and an experience. N. Engl. J. Med. 210:748, 1934.
5. Magoun, H: The Walking Brain. Charles C Thomas, Springfield, Ill., 1963.
6. Oxbury, J., Campbell, D., and Oxbury, S.: Unilateral spatial neglect and impairment of spatial analysis and perception. Brain 97:551, 1974.
7. Watson, R., Heilman, K., Miller, B., and King, F.: Neglect after mesencephalic reticular formation lesions. Neurology 24:294, 1974.

CHAPTER 4

Behavioral Observations

Before beginning formal mental status testing, it is important to make specific and systematic observations of the patient's appearance, mood, and behavior. Subsequent sections of the examination deal primarily with changes in cognitive ability that can be objectively evaluated. This chapter is concerned with the changes in emotions and behavior that may be seen with organic brain disease. A careful observation of behavior is important because (1) there are specific behavioral syndromes that correspond to well recognized neurologic disease entities (e.g., the frontal lobe syndrome), (2) such observations provide crucial data to aid in the differential diagnosis between organic and functional disorders, (3) the results of more formal cognitive testing must be interpreted in the context of basic behavioral data (e.g., depression may hamper cooperation and secondarily test performance), and (4) a significant behavioral disturbance may dramatically interfere with subsequent formal testing (e.g., a patient in an organic confusional state will perform poorly on memory testing because of inattention). Sufficient information regarding behavior is not always available from a short period of direct observation and must be obtained from history provided by family members or other reliable observers.

The primary purpose of this section is to provide a formal framework to assist the examiner in systematically observing behavior. Within this general framework, certain alterations in behavior have particular diagnostic significance and must be examined in detail. The discussions of behavior in this chapter are primarily concerned with the identification and description of organic disease and its effects. Extensive discussions of behavior from a psychiatric viewpoint are included in all major psychiatric texts (e.g., Stevenson and Sheppe,[15] Detre and Kupfer[7]).

EVALUATION

History

There are certain elements in the patient's medical history that are of particular importance in evaluating mental status. The following outline is provided to assist the examiner in recording these data.

1. Family history
   a. Neurologic or psychiatric disease in another family member
   b. Familial neurologic disease (e.g., Huntington's chorea)
   c. Familial predilection for a particular disease process that may involve the central nervous system (e.g., hypertension and stroke)
2. Birth and developmental history
   a. Brain damage from birth
   b. Developmental delays
      1) Motor
      2) Language
      3) Intellectual
      4) Academic
3. Past history
   a. Previous neurologic disease
   b. Central nervous system infections
   c. Significant head trauma
   d. Seizures
4. Description of present illness
   a. Nature of onset
   b. Duration of the illness
   c. Description of behavioral change associated with illness
5. Other relevant neurobehavioral data
   a. Memory difficulty
   b. Difficulty with geographic orientation (i.e., getting lost)
   c. Recent onset of reading, writing, or calculating difficulties
   d. Attention and concentration problems
   e. Recent onset of language problems
   f. Unusual or bizarre behavior (e.g., nocturnal wanderings or paranoia)
6. Educational and vocational history
   a. Highest school grade attained
   b. Adequacy as a student (grade failures)
   c. Vocation
      1) Type of jobs
      2) Frequency of job changes
      3) Recent problems with job

Physical Appearance

Many patients with either brain disease or functional disorders show characteristic patterns of physical appearance. Classic examples range from that of the patient with organic unilateral neglect with a total lack of attention to dress, care (e.g., shaving and washing), and even presence of one side of the body to that of the obsessive-compulsive neurotic patient who may be scrupulously dressed and groomed, and unnecessarily fastidious in matters relating to cleanliness and manner. Obvious neurologic signs such as hemiplegia or chorea will not be specifically mentioned; it is important to realize that the mental status examination is but one part of the complete neurologic evaluation. The following aspects of appearance should be systematically reviewed and noted.

1. General appearance
   a. Description data
      1) Age
      2) Height
      3) Weight
   b. General impression of appearance
      1) Appearance for chronological age
      2) Posture
      3) Facial expression
      4) Eye contact
2. Personal cleanliness
   a. Skin
   b. Hair
   c. Nails
   d. Teeth
   e. Beard
   f. Indications of unilateral neglect
3. Habits of dress
   a. Type of clothing
   b. Cleanliness of clothing
   c. Sloppiness in dressing
   d. Overly fastidious in dress and grooming
   e. Indications of unilateral neglect
4. Motor activity
   a. Level of general activity
      1) Placid vs. tense
      2) Hyperkinetic vs. hypokinetic
   b. Abnormal posturing
      1) Tics

2) Facial grimaces
3) Bizarre gestures
4) Other involuntary movements

Mood and General Emotional Status

By mood, we refer to the prevailing and conscious emotional feeling during the period of the mental status examination. Moods tend to be more persistent and less intense than specific emotional responses to particular situations or other stimuli. Emotional status is a more general behavioral response which may be evaluated through direct observation of the patient's behavior during the examination. Both certain organic brain diseases (e.g., frontal lobe disease) and psychiatric conditions may be distinguished by rather characteristic disturbances of mood and emotional status. Obviously, disturbances of mood and emotional status will affect performance on subsequent portions of the mental status examination and will also have a significant impact upon the patient's life in general. Accordingly, a careful and systematic review of the following behavioral components is important for the comprehensive mental status examination. This is not intended as a complete and definitive psychiatric examination, but rather provides a framework for the brief assessment of emotional status. This assessment is necessary both for the identification of organically based behavior change and for the initial differentiation of functional and organic disease. Those readers desiring a more comprehensive overview of the psychiatric interpretation of mood and emotional status disturbances may refer to any comprehensive psychiatric text.

1. Mood
   a. Mood normal to the situation
   b. Feeling of sadness (hopelessness, grief, or loss)
   c. Feelings of elation (inappropriate optimism or boastfulness)
   d. Apathy and lack of concern
   e. Constantness or fluctuations in mood
   f. Inappropriate mood: expressed effect is not consistent with the content of his thought
2. Emotional status
   a. Degree of cooperation with the examiner
   b. Anxiety
   c. Depression
   d. Suspiciousness
   e. Anger
   f. Specific inappropriate emotional responses to particular situations
   g. Reality testing
      1) Delusions (false beliefs)

2) Illusions (misperceptions of real stimuli)
3) Hallucinations
4) Paranoid thinking
h. Indications of specific neurotic symptoms
1) Phobias
2) Chronic anxiety
3) Obsessive-compulsive thinking and/or behavior
4) Depression
i. Abnormalities in language or speech
1) Neologisms: (personal formation of a new word without real meaning except to the patient)
2) Flight of ideas in thinking and speaking
3) Loose associations in thinking and speaking

Additional Diagnostic Procedures and Techniques

Diseases of the frontal lobes may be difficult to evaluate clinically because of the relative absence of clearcut cognitive changes with lesions of this area.[1,16] There are, however, some behavior changes which are characteristic of dysfunction in this area of the brain and some specific clinical tests which can readily be administered at the bedside to assess the integrity of this area.

Alternating Sequences—Visual Pattern Completion

Directions. Present the patient with the following visual patterns on individual sheets of white paper (see Fig. 4-1). Tell him to reproduce the stimulus figure and then to continue the alternating sequence. Give additional elaboration of the directions to ensure that the patient has understood the nature of the test. Do not correct his errors or provide additional cues after he begins the task.

Scoring. Patients with intact motor and sensory systems should be capable of completing the above sequences without error. A loss of the sequence or indications of perseveration in the reproduction of sequences are suggestive of a loss in the ability to move from one motor movement to another and an inability to shift sets efficiently. This may be indicative of frontal lobe dysfunction. Examples of common errors are shown in Figure 4-2.

Alternating Motor Patterns

Directions. This test consists of a series of changes in hand position. They have been adapted from Luria[10] and are described in greater detail in that source.

27

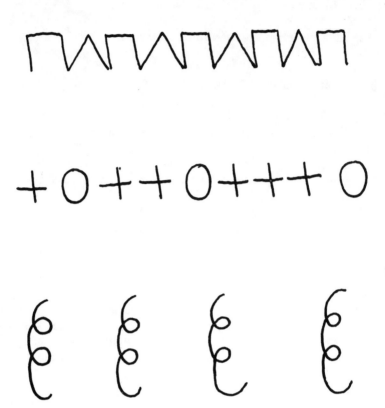

FIGURE 4-1.   Test items for Visual Pattern Completion Test.

1. Fist-Palm-Side Test

Tell the patient to repeatedly hit the top of the desk, first with his fist, then with his open palm, and then with the side of his hand. Demonstrate the task once and then tell the patient to perform the task until told to stop. Performance for 15-20 seconds should suffice to assess the adequacy of these alternating movements.

2. Fist-Ring Test

Instruct the patient to extend his arm several times, first with his hand in a fist and then with the thumb and forefinger opposed to form a ring. Demonstrate the action and then tell the patient to perform the action. With successive extensions of the arm, he alternates between these two positions.

3. Reciprocol Coordination Test

This is an alternation test utilizing both hands. Initially the patient places both hands on the desk, one in a fist and one with the fingers extended palm down. Tell the patient to rapidly alternate the position of

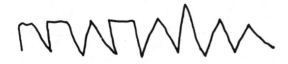

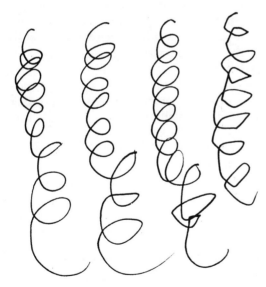

FIGURE 4-2.   Common errors in Visual Pattern Completion Test.

the two hands (simultaneously extending the fingers of one hand while making a fist with the other). Demonstrate the nature of the task.

Scoring. Normal patients should have no difficulty in easily mastering these alternating sequences after one or two attempts.[10] Accordingly, any appreciable disrupton of smooth performance on these tasks is indicative of dysfunction of the premotor areas of the cerebral cortex.

Anatomy and Clinical Implications

There are several distinct clinical entities that are recognized primarily through behavioral observation rather than by specific cognitive testing. These syndromes involve defects in mood and emotional reaction more than alternations in cognition. The diagnosis, therefore, is made by systematic behavioral observation.

Acute Confusional State

The most common of these behavioral syndromes seen in a general hospital population is the acute confusional state. The terms "toxic delirium," "acute brain syndrome," "organic brain syndrome with psychosis," "acute exogenous reaction," and "toxic encephalopathy" have all been employed to describe this state. The acute confusional state has a characteristic group of behavioral and historic findings. The onset of symptoms is usually acute (appearing over a period of hours or days), the patients are inattentive and produce incoherent conversation which drifts from the central point, they are inconsistent in reporting recent events (e.g., the patient may tell the examiner that he has just come back from a walk with a friend when in fact he has been in his hospital bed for the entire day), and they often demonstrate fluctuations in their level of consciousness. Hallucinations, usually visual, and agitation are often present. Patients who are grossly confusional may be severely agitated, shout incoherently, and may require restraints to prevent them from disrupting IV's, urinary catheters, and other apparatus. Conversely, some patients may appear superficially normal, but on systematic examination will demonstrate mild degrees of inattention, disorientation, difficulties in carrying out a coherent conversation, and upon specific questioning may admit to nocturnal hallucinations and delusions. The individual patient's confusion is not stable and tends to wax and wane during the day and night. At night when environmental stimuli are reduced, the confusion and agitation become accentuated.

The confusional state is a very important abnormal behavioral pattern to recognize because it represents an acute medical state rather than a psychiatric condition. Metabolic imbalance, toxic reaction to drugs, sepsis, increased intracranial pressure, or withdrawal reactions are the most common etiologies. Elderly patients are the most sensitive to subtle changes in homeostasis and frequently become confused postoperatively when electrolytes are slightly out of balance and strong analgesics have been administered for pain. Patients in early heart, pulmonary, or hepatic failure may also show confusion.

Although psychiatrists are often consulted to see these patients because of their abnormal behavior, all such conditions require primary medical treatment. However, even with the administration of proper medical treatment, the confusional state may linger for many days until intracellular balance and general synaptic function are restored. During this period, tranquilizers may be used to calm the patient's agitation.

The confusional state does not usually result from focal brain lesions, but is rather a reflection of widespread cortical and subcortical neuronal dysfunction. The cortical dysfunction causes an alteration in the content of consciousness, whereas involvement of the ascending activating system leads to the disturbances of basic arousal.

In the patient with a confusional state, further mental status testing will be invalid. Inattention plus general cortical dysfunction does not allow the patient to perform adequately on memory, abstract reasoning, or even writing tasks.[5] Since the confusion is often slow to clear, definitive mental status testing should be postponed. If the full test is done while the patient is confused, a misdiagnosis of dementia can easily be inadvertently made. As the changes in the brain are physiologic rather than structural, the patient's level of functioning should eventually return to premorbid levels.

Although the acute onset of inattention, agitation, fluctuating levels of alertness, incoherent speech and train of thought, and visual hallucinations is most often due to a medical condition, the differential diagnosis must include consideration of various functional psychiatric disorders such as acute schizophrenic episode, severe anxiety or panic state, agitated depression, and mania.

The differentiation between the acute organic confusional states and acute severe functional disorders is difficult, but may usually be accurately made with data provided from the patient's medical and psychiatric history, the medical examination, and some aspects of the mental status examination. Alterations in the level of consciousness are almost invariably associated with organic brain disease. Visual hallucinations are more typically seen in the organic patient, whereas auditory hallucinations are more common in functional psychoses. Systematized delusional systems are infrequent in the patient with an acute confusional state. In any case where the etiology is unclear, the psychiatrist, neurologist, and primary physician should work closely together to conduct a full evaluation.

Frontal Lobe Syndrome

Patients with bilateral frontal lobe disease will not typically show dramatic cognitive deficits on formal mental status testing, but will often demonstrate specific personality changes. The most common features of the frontal lobe personality are apathy, both during examination and toward work and family; euphoria with a tendency toward jocularity; irritability that is short lived; and social inappropriateness.[9] Some frontal lobe patients are predominantly apathetic; they sit around and show little interest in any aspect of their environment. In such patients, the apathy is sometimes misconstrued as depression and lengthy expensive and ineffective psychiatric treatment can be undertaken if a careful neurologic examination is not done. Although these patients are primarily apathetic, they may become very irritable and argumentative for short periods of time when sufficiently stressed. Conversely, other patients are primarily loud, jocular, inappropriately intrusive, or socially aggressive. Because of their outgoing behavior, such patients may give the initial impression of interest and productivity. However, this emotional dysinhibition and euphoria does not result in constructive activity. In general, the patient with frontal damage has lost both interest in his environment and also his productive social drive. Such patients often fail to maintain job performance, normal family relations, or even personal cleanliness. Since the frontal lobes are the areas of the brain in which reason and emotion interact,[11] bilateral damage may leave the individual with apathy, unchecked emotions, and an intellect without social and emotional guidance.

The following are two clinical examples of patients with frontal lobe syndromes. Mrs. L. is a 58-year-old housewife who was brought to the hospital by her daughter with a one year history of decreasing interest in caring for her house and personal needs. The patient lived alone in a rural area with few neighbors. The daughter during an infrequent visit had noticed a change in her mother's behavior characterized by a lack of interest in conversation, unkempt appearance, a lack of concern about family affairs, and total neglect of personal and household cleanliness. Neighbors had noticed that the patient had discontinued attending church, did very little shopping, and no longer made social visits. Upon examination at hospital admission, Mrs. L. was awake, yet markedly apathetic. She offered no spontaneous conversation and answered all questions with only single word responses. She had a slow shuffling gait and had several episodes of incontinence. Neurodiagnostic evaluation (C.A.T. scan) demonstrated a large frontal cyst. Surgical exploration with drainage produced a marked behavioral reversal. Within two weeks, the patient was walking well, conversing spontaneously, and was no longer apathetic or incontinent.

Mrs. L. represented the primarily apathetic variation of the frontal lobe syndrome.

Conversely, the following is a case which demonstrates dysinhibition, social inappropriateness, and jocularity which may be associated with the underlying apathy in some cases of this syndrome. Mr. N. is a 65-year-old male who was brought to the hospital by his wife. Her chief complaint was that her husband's mind was deranged. The wife stated that her husband had always been a great joker but had used proper social restraint until about four or five years ago. At that time, he began to show excessive candor in his remarks to friends and acquaintances. His usual outgoing personality gave way to flippancy and arrogance. His prior restraint was decreased and he approached each social situation with an almost aggressive egotism, with much showing off and boasting.

Over the past years, he has lost regard for his personal cleaniness; bathing and shaving only at his wife's behest. His wife also reported that his memory has started to fail and that he confabulates on occasion. Recently, she bought a new lawn mower and brought it home with the handle disassembled. She asked him to put the handle together and put it on the mower, but he was unable to do so.

In the last few months, he has become quite agitated and somewhat paranoid. He wanders around the neighborhood and often tells strangers fantastic tales, the last being that he was an undercover agent for the FBI. His judgment in other matters has also deteriorated. The last time he drove the car, he went through a stop sign and joked about it with his wife. These last events prompted his referral to the hospital. Examination revealed an inattentive, restless, socially inappropriate man who was physically unkempt with uncombed hair, uncut finger and toe nails, and messy clothes. He exhibited some paranoia, asking if the medicine (Thorazine) was some sort of poison; several times during the exam he attempted to leave the room and was obviously agitated. His thought processes were extremely concrete and he performed poorly on virtually all aspects of the mental status examination. During the hospital period he became quite upset and irritable, especially at night, and even was somewhat aggressive with several nurses. The C.A.T. scan revealed frontotemporal atrophy with greatly enlarged frontal horns and widened sulci. The presumptive diagnosis in this case was Pick's disease. This represents a type of dementia that frequently presents as a frontal lobe syndrome.

If the behavioral manifestations of the frontal lobe syndrome are present, the following neurologic diseases should be considered in the differential diagnosis: (1) tumors—subfrontal meningiomas, pituitary adenomas, or primary brain tumors, (2) head trauma with frontal contusions, (3) Pick's disease, (4) general paresis, (5) communicating hydrocephalus, and (6) Huntington's chorea. Any patient with extensive cortical disease (e.g., late Alzheimer's disease, multiple cortical infarcts, or traumatic or postinfectious encephalopathy) will show some of the behavior changes seen in the frontal lobe patient. However, such patients also show evidence of severe cognitive dysfunction and other indications of involvement of other brain areas.

Temporal Lobe Epilepsy

Some patients with chronic temporal lobe epilepsy develop characteristic changes in emotional behavior. Some of these changes are associated with the seizure itself (ictal phenomena), while others represent more permanent changes in personality (interictal phenomena). Among the more common ictal phenomena are déjà vu experiences, transient visual or auditory hallucinations, feelings of depersonalization, fear, anger, delusions or illusions, sexual feelings, and paranoia. The interictal behavior changes are more significant because they represent a chronic change in personality. Many patients demonstrate a global hyposexuality which is frequently manifested by a total lack of interest in sex.[4] With this decrease in sexual interest is a concomitant increase in social aggressiveness. This combination of behavior changes seems to represent an imbalance in limbic functions secondary to the irritative focus in the medial temporal lobe. Some temporal lobe seizure patients develop abnormal sexual behavior when their seizures are not well controlled. This abnormal sexuality will revert to normal with the establishment of adequate medical control.[2,3] An increase in religious interest is seen in many patients and in rare cases actual fervent religious conversion has been reported during periods of increased epileptiform activity in the temporal lobe.[8] This religiosity is often coupled with paranoia. The abnormal behavior change seen in patients with chronic temporal lobe epilepsy varies widely. There is a higher than expected incidence of schizophreniform psychosis in such patients.[14]

Any patient presenting with the behavior changes described above should be evaluated for temporal lobe epilepsy; although these behavioral abnormalities are usually seen only in patients with well documented chronic seizures.

Apathy versus Depression

The differentiation between apathy and depression is a difficult, but extremely important, distinction to make. By apathy we refer to a disorder of mood which is characterized by a significant indifference to the external stimuli, and a marked emotional blunting. This is a behavioral symptom which can be seen with large bilateral frontal lobe lesions, large right hemisphere lesions, and bilateral brain disease. Apathy is a common symptom of organic brain disease, although it may also be seen in functional depression. The observation of apathy does not justify a diagnosis of depression. If apathy is the only symptom of depression present, a careful search for an organic etiology should be undertaken. The devastating effect of misdiagnosing depression in an apathetic patient with a frontal lobe tumor is obvious.

Patients with primary depression may appear demented to the inexperienced examiner because their apathy results in impaired memory, abstract reasoning, and concentration. This reduced cognitive performance associated with functional illness has been classified as a pseudodementia.[12,13] Similarly, the patient with agitated depression will perform poorly on mental status tests because of reduced attention. With appropriate treatment of the psychiatric condition, the patient's mental status will revert to premorbid levels. The misdiagnosing of depression as dementia is as egregious an error as diagnosing a frontal lobe tumor as depression.

Denial and Neglect

Some patients develop a striking degree of denial of their illness as a direct result of a brain lesion. This form of denial does not seem to be the result of a strengthening of the psychologic defense mechanisms, but is a more basic and unusual organic behavior change. Clinically there is a spectrum of denial and neglect syndromes ranging from explicit denial of illness as the most severe behavioral abnormality to mild suppression of stimulation on one side of the body during bilateral simultaneous stimulation (inattention or extinction). The patient with gross denial may deny total cortical blindness (Anton's syndrome) or a severe hemiplegia (anosognosia). When asked about his illness, such a patient may say that he is in the hospital for tests to evaluate mild joint pain or some similar benign condition. Some patients state that they are not really in a hospital at all, but merely in a rest facility or hotel (reduplication of place or paramnesia). The patient remains steadfast in his denial even when his paralyzed arm is demonstrated to him. He will often make elaborate excuses of fatigue when asked to perform with the paralyzed limb (confabulation) and on occasion will even claim that the weak arm is not his (reduplication of body parts). The hemiplegic patient who denies weakness is a great problem in rehabilitation because he is unaware of his weakness and tends to fall repeatedly.

Some patients do not demonstrate frank denial, but do have a dramatic neglect of one side of the body. Such patients may shave only one side of the face, use only one sleeve of their robe, and fail to use one side of the body even though paralysis is not present. These patients also neglect one half of the extrapersonal environment even in the absence of a visual field defect. For example, the patient may fail to respond to a visitor who approaches him on his involved side. The patient may also show neglect

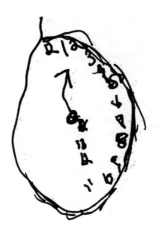

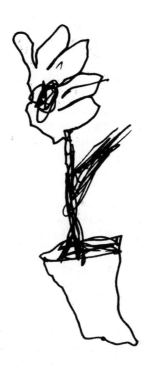

FIGURE 4-3.   Examples of neglect on drawing test.

on drawing tasks. Examples of this type of neglect are shown in Figure 4-3.

The most subtle form of neglect is an inattention to one side of the body when both sides are simultaneously stimulated. This tendency to suppress or extinguish the stimuli on the involved side is discussed in detail in the previous chapter.

The lesion that most frequently causes the denial and neglect syndromes is a nondominant hemisphere lesion, most frequently vascular in etiology.[6] A specific lesion locus within the right hemisphere has not yet been established. Subcortical as well as cortical structures may be involved. Gross explicit denial is an uncommon behavioral finding that is most frequently seen during the acute stages of a vascular accident, is frequently associated with a degree of confusion, and may only be seen in patients with predisposing personality characteristics. Unilateral neglect may be seen as a chronic effect of parietal lesions, predominantly in the nondominant hemisphere. The actual neuropsychologic and neurophysiologic mechanisms underlying these syndromes are not completely understood. Patients with frontal lobe disease and patients in confusional states may also show evidence of denial. The reader is referred to Weinstein and Kahn[17] for a clinical review of this problem with case studies.

SUMMARY

Organic brain lesions may cause a multiplicity of behavioral syndromes, some of which are characteristic of specific clinical conditions. The examiner must be prepared to make a systematic evaluation of the patient's behavior and be able to recognize the major neurobehavioral syndromes.

REFERENCES

1. Black, W.: Cognitive deficits in patients with unilateral war-related frontal lobe lesions. J. Clin. Psychol. 32:307, 1976.
2. Blumer, D.: Transsexualism, sexual dysfunction, and temporal lobe disorder, in Green, R., and Money, J. (eds.): Transsexualism and Sexual Reassignment. Johns Hopkins Press, Baltimore, 1969, pp. 213-219.
3. Blumer, D.: Hypersexual episodes in temporal lobe epilepsy. Am. J. Psychiat. 126:1099, 1970.
4. Blumer, D., and Walker, A. E.: Sexual behavior in temporal lobe epilepsy. Arch. Neurol. 16:37, 1967.
5. Chédru, F., and Geschwind, N.: Writing disturbances in acute confusional states. Neuropsychol. 10:343, 1972.
6. Critchley, M.: The Parietal Lobes. Edward Arnold and Company, London, 1953.
7. Detre, T. P., and Kupfer, D. J.: Psychiatric history and mental status examination, in Freedman, A., Kaplan, H., and Sadock, B. (eds.): Comprehensive Textbook of Psychiatry, Vol. 1. Williams and Wilkins, Baltimore, 1975, pp. 724-735.

8. Dewhurst, K., and Beard, A. W.: Sudden religious conversions in temporal lobe epilepsy. Br. J. Psychiat. 117:497, 1970.
9. Hecaen, H., and Albert, M. L.: Disorders of mental functioning related to frontal lobe pathology, in Benson, D. F., and Blummer, P. (eds.). Psychiatric Aspects of Neurologic Disease. Grune and Stratton, New York, 1975, pp. 137-149.
10. Luria, A. R.: Traumatic Aphasia. Mouton and Company, The Hague, 1970.
11. Nauta, W. J. H.: The problem of the frontal lobe, a reinterpretation. J. Psychiat. Res. 8:167, 1971.
12. Nott, P. N., and Fleminger, J. J.: Presenile dementia: The difficulties of early diagnosis. Acta Psychiat. Scand. 51:210, 1975.
13. Post, F.: Dementia, depression and pseudo-dementia, in Benson, D. F., and Blummer, P. (eds.): Psychiatric Aspects of Neurologic Disease. Grune and Stratton, New York, 1975, pp. 99-120.
14. Slater, E., Beard, A. W., and Glithero, E.: The schizophrenia-like psychoses of epilepsy. Br. J. Psychiat. 109:95, 1963.
15. Stevenson, I., and Sheppe, W. M.: The psychiatric examination, in Arieti, S. (ed.): American Handbook of Psychiatry, Vol. 1. Basic Books, New York, pp. 215-234, 1959.
16. Teuber, H. L.: The riddle of frontal lobe function in man, in Warren, J., and Alert, K. (eds.): The Frontal Granular Cortex and Behavior. McGraw-Hill, New York, 1964, pp. 410-444.
17. Weinstein, E. A., and Kahn, R. L.: Denial of Illness. Charles C Thomas, Springfield, Ill., 1955.

CHAPTER 5

Language

Language is the basic tool of human communication. It is crucial in assessing most cognitive abilities; therefore its integrity must be established early in the course of mental status testing. Language disturbances are commonly seen in patients with focal or diffuse brain disease; in fact demonstration of a specific language disturbance is pathognomonic of brain damage. Language disturbances have been well studied and a number of distinct clinical neuroanatomic syndromes have been described. These are of importance to the clinician because of the relationship of specific language syndromes with neuroanatomic lesions. The ability to communicate with language is critical to the patient and any disruption of this ability will result in a significant handicap in his day to day living. If deficits are found in the language system, subsequent evaluation of cognitive factors such as verbal memory, proverb interpretation, and oral calculations becomes difficult if not impossible.

The examiner must develop a systematic approach to language and become acquainted with the various classic language syndromes. Cerebral vascular accidents (strokes), brain tumors, trauma, and other lesions give rise to a variety of language disturbances. These disturbances are not always easily characterized by the casual examiner. A familiarity with testing and the patterns of language disruption will make the aphasias, alexias, and agraphias more understandable.

TERMINOLOGY

Dysarthria refers to a specific disorder of articulation in which basic language—grammar and word choice—is intact. Patients with pure dysarthria produce distorted speech sounds that cannot be accurately transcribed by a listener. The speech can be unintelligible and may not resemble English speech sounds.

Dysprosody is an interruption of speech melody. Speech inflection and rhythm are disturbed. The resulting speech production can be monotonal, halting, and can at times mimic a foreign accent.

Buccofacial or oral apraxia is the inability to carry out skilled movements of the face and speech apparatus in the presence of normal comprehension, muscle strength, and coordination. When asked to show how he would blow out a match, the apraxic patient may have difficulty approximating a pucker, inhale instead of exhale, exhale vigorously without puckering his lips, or merely say the word "blow." Any of these errors would be classified as apraxic.

Aphasia is a true language disturbance in which the patient produces errors of grammar and word choice. The basic aphasic defect is in higher integrative language processing, although articulation and praxic errors may be present. Aphasia usually refers to a loss of language after brain damage, but the term developmental aphasia is sometimes used when a child has a specific delay in language acquisition disproportionate to general cognitive development.

Alexia is the term used to describe a loss of reading ability in a previously literate person with adequate visual acuity. Alexia does not refer only to a total loss of reading ability, but to any level of disturbance in reading. Alexia is not synonymous with dyslexia. This term refers to a specific developmental learning disorder of children who have normal intelligence, yet experience unusual difficulty in learning to read.

Agraphia is an acquired disturbance in writing. It refers specifically to errors of language and not to problems with the actual formation of letters. Agraphia does not refer to poor handwriting secondary to any cause.

EVALUATION

The evaluation of the language system should be carried out in an orderly fashion. Specific attention must be paid to spontaneous speech, comprehension, repetition, and naming. Reading and writing should be assessed after verbal language has been evaluated. A short period of systematic testing can usually identify and roughly characterize an aphasic deficit. The aphasic patient is always agraphic and frequently is alexic, accordingly, in these cases the testing of reading and writing may be abbreviated. In the nonaphasic patient, reading and writing should be fully evaluated as alexia and/or agraphia may be seen in isolation. Language testing can be very comprehensive, and for further information the interested examiner is referred to the test batteries listed in Appendix 1.

Handedness

Handedness and cerebral dominance for language are closely allied, therefore, the patient's handedness should be determined prior to language testing. First, ask the patient whether he is right or left handed. Many natural left handers have been taught to write with the right hand. Accordingly, observation of the hand used for writing may not be an accurate reflection of natural handedness. Next, ask the patient which hand he uses to hold a knife, throw a ball, stir coffee, and flip a coin. Also ask him if he has any tendency to use the opposite hand for any skilled movement. In addition, a family history of left handedness or ambidexterity is important since cerebral dominance for language is significantly influenced by heredity. There is a spectrum of handedness ranging from strong right handedness to strong left handedness. Handedness should be reported as follows: strong right handedness, weak right handedness, ambidexterity, weak left handedness, or strong left handedness.

Spontaneous Speech

The first step in language testing is to listen carefully to the patient's spontaneous speech. If he offers none, certain open ended questions should be asked to stimulate speech production. It is wise to ask relatively uncomplicated questions such as "Tell me why you are in the hospital," or "Tell me a bit about your work." This type of general conversational question affords the patient a familiar topic and usually elicits his best efforts. In contrast, questions requiring a mere "yes" or "no" answer will not provide sufficient speech output for evaluation. Pictures may be used to stimulate speech. However, they can restrict language output because of unfamiliarity and the limited speech response possible to a specific stimulus.

Several observations must be made while listening to the patient's spontaneous speech. First, is speech output present? Second, is the speech dysarthric or dysprosodic? Third, is there evidence of specific aphasic errors? The most obviously abnormal output is the total lack of any speech. These patients may make some vocalizations, but no meaningful linguistic utterances. This reduced output may be due to a severe dysarthria, apraxia (buccofacial), or a true aphasia. Next in severity is a specific aphasic disorder characterized by stereotyped output in which the patient repeats the same utterance in response to each question. The utterance is usually a nonsense word like "bica, bica" or "a dis, a dis, a dis." Patients with very restricted output can, however, often surprise the naive examiner by producing well articulated curse words or short phrases under emotional stress.

Aphasic language production is characterized by errors of grammatical structure, difficulty in word finding, and the presence of word substitutions (paraphasias). One common type of aphasic speech pattern has been classified as nonfluent.[1,7] Nonfluent output is sparse, effortful, contains primarily nouns (substantive words), is agrammatic, and contains frequent word finding pauses. For instance, the nonfluent patient describing winter weather might say, "ah, ah, chold . . . snow . . . freezing . . . ah, ah . . . cold." At the other end of the spectrum of fluency is a group of aphasics who produce an easily flowing speech that is remarkably empty of content and contains many abnormal words (paraphasias). Paraphasias are words that are either substitutions for the correct word (e.g., "I drove home in my *pen*") or contain substituted syllables (e.g., "I drove home in my *lar*"). The complete word substitution ("pen" for "car") is a verbal or semantic paraphasia. The syllable substitution ("lar" for "car") is a phonemic or literal paraphasia. A third variety of paraphasia is the neologistic (new word) paraphasia which is a completely non-English word substitution (e.g., "I drove home in my *strub*"). Paraphasic speech is an easily recognizable speech pattern. The output is fluent, and is characterized by normal or excessive rate of word production, often with a distinct press of speech (rapid pressure to speak). Content words (nouns and verbs) are lacking and in contradistinction to nonfluent output, small grammatical words such as articles, conjunctions, and interjections prevail. The nouns and verbs are often paraphasic. Because of the difficulty in producing nouns, word finding pauses may interrupt the easy flow of speech. A fluent aphasic describing a picture of a man following a shipwreck said the following, "It is a . . . I can see it . . . It is near a cold and he has a . . . actually what has happened is part of a . . . The rest of it there is a man right here and he is cold being out there." Occasionally, the language of the aphasic contains so many paraphasic errors that the discourse is virtually unintelligible and is difficult to follow. The term jargon aphasia is used for this heavily paraphasic, but fluent speech.

The expressive language of many aphasics cannot be strictly classified according to the above categories, but, rather, is a mixture of types. The primary goal for the student evaluating a brain damaged patient is to recognize that the language production is aphasic. With experience, the examiner will be able to accurately classify the patient's language output. The classification of language output often gives important information as to the locus of the brain lesion. The classification of an aphasia does not rest upon the output characteristics alone; a full language evaluation is always indicated.

Comprehension

Comprehension of spoken language is the next step in the comprehensive language evaluation. Language comprehension must be assessed in a structured fashion and without reliance upon the patient's ability to produce speech. The most common error in assessment is asking the patient to answer general or open ended questions. A question requiring the patient to construct a complex verbal answer tests the integrity of the entire language system and not verbal comprehension in isolation. To fully evaluate the patient's aphasia, each aspect of language must be individually tested. Comprehensive testing should require the minimum verbal response necessary for the patient to demonstrate that he has understood the examiner. For example, asking the patient to answer the question, "What was the weather like in January?" does not assess language comprehension in isolation as does asking, "Is it snowing out today?"

We use two methods of testing comprehension: pointing commands and questions that can be answered with a yes or no response. Pointing to single objects in the room, body parts, or articles collected from the examiner's pockets (e.g., coins, comb, pencil, key, etc.) is an excellent way to quantify single word comprehension. This task may be increased in complexity by requiring that the patient point to an increasing sequence of objects. Start by asking the patient to point to single objects. Increase the number of objects until the patient consistently fails. The patient of average intelligence without aphasia should succeed in pointing to four objects or more. The aphasic with comprehension difficulty may be able to accurately point to one or two items, therefore, it is important to continue testing until a point of consistent failure is reached. This test provides an evaluation of single word comprehension, auditory retention, and sequence memory. For clarity, the results should be recorded as, "Patient successfully pointed to two items." Many patients will make errors of sequence, while others will remember only the first or last item presented.

Next a series of simple and complex questions requiring yes or no answers should be asked. For example: "Is this a hotel?" "Is it raining today?" "Do you eat breakfast before dinner?" Material may be as simple or complex as necessary. Before testing, be sure that the patient can reliably indicate "yes" and "no." Many patients will confuse these two terms and be unable to accurately speak or nod appropriately. Also, it is important to ask at least six questions as correct responses can occur by chance alone 50 per cent of the time with yes/no questions. Correct answers should alternate from yes to no randomly because brain damaged patients tend to perseverate. It is not uncommon for a patient to answer "yes" to ten questions consecutively without knowing the correct answer to any of the questions.

Many clinicians test comprehension by asking patients to carry out motor commands such as, "Show me how to light a cigarette," "Stick out your tongue," or "Indicate by raising the appropriate number of fingers on your right hand, the position in the alphabet of the first letter in the name of the city in which we are." (answer: Two, for a major northeastern city where this question has actually been used to test for aphasia.) If the patient correctly carries out such commands, he has certainly understood them; however, many aphasic patients have significant apraxia and fail to follow the command because of a high level motor problem and not because of poor verbal comprehension. For this reason, verbal commands must be used with caution.

Repetition

Repetition of spoken language is linguistically and to some extent anatomically a distinct function. Therefore, it is clinically relevant to test it specifically. Additionally, in aphasia, repetition may be spared or involved in isolation. Repetition is a complex process which can be affected by impaired auditory processing, disturbed speech production, or disconnection between the receptive and expressive language areas.

Testing should be done with material of ascending difficulty. Start with single monosyllabic words and proceed to complex sentences. The following list of items is suggested to provide a range of difficulty. Ask the patient to repeat the word or sentence after the examiner.

1. Ball
2. Help
3. Airplane
4. Hospital
5. Mississippi River
6. The little boy went home.
7. We all went over there together.
8. Let's go downtown for ice cream.
9. The fat short boy dropped the china vase.
10. Each fight readied the boxer for the championship bout.

The examiner must listen for paraphasias, grammatical errors, omissions, and additions, as well as obvious failures to approximate the examples given.

Naming and Word Finding

The ability to name objects is one of the earliest acquired and most basic language functions. It is also almost invariably disturbed in every type of aphasia.[10] Word finding difficulty is closely related to impaired naming ability (anomia) and refers to a reduced availability of the nouns and verbs used in spontaneous speech. Specific word finding problems can be detected by listening to the aphasic patient's spontaneous speech. Asking the patient to describe a picture containing objects and actions will dramatize the word finding defect. Anomia is best assessed by confrontation naming. In confrontation naming, the examiner points to a variety of objects and asks the patient to name them. The examiner should select from 10 to 20 items. Several categories of objects should be used (colors, body parts, room objects, articles of clothing, and parts of objects). Various categories are chosen as some aphasic patients have a curious inability to name objects in a specific category while maintaining adequate ability to name objects in other categories. Since the disruption of naming has varying degrees of severity, it is important to use uncommon (low frequency of usage) items as well as common (high frequency) items. For example, "nose," "arm," and "floor" are common, high frequency words, whereas "watch crystal," "shin," and "coat lapel" are uncommon low frequency words. Many aphasics will be able to quickly and accurately name common words, only to show great hesitancy, paraphasia, and circumlocution with low frequency or uncommon objects.

The following 20 items listed in ascending order of difficulty (frequency of usage) are suggested to evaluate naming ability. The examiner should note that the labels for parts of objects are less frequently used in expressive speech and, accordingly, most aphasics will have relatively more difficulty with this category. With experience, the examiner may develop his personal repertoire of items tailored to his own office and patient population.

TABLE 5-1. Objects for confrontation naming in ascending order of difficulty by category

Colors	Body parts
Red	Eye
Blue	Leg
Yellow	Teeth
Pink	Thumb
Purple	Knuckles

Clothing and room objects	Parts of objects
Door	Watch stem (winder)
Watch	Coat lapel
Shoe	Watch crystal
Shirt	Sole of shoe
Ceiling	Buckle of belt

Reading

Reading ability is one of the few aspects of mental status testing which is strictly related to educational experience. It is important, therefore, to determine the patient's educational background before testing reading. Having demonstrated an alexia (reading deficit) in a patient, only to discover that he has had but three years of formal education is merely to document his illiteracy.

Both reading comprehension and reading aloud should be tested. Both are usually defective in the same patient, but either can be disturbed in isolation. Testing reading in the aphasic should begin with short single words, then phrases, sentences, and finally paragraphs. Single words should refer to objects, while phrases and sentences should demand a yes-no response. First have the patient read the item aloud and then have him indicate comprehension by pointing to the object or saying or nodding "yes" or "no." For example, if the patient read the sentence. "The boy and girl walked in the snow," the examiner could ask, "Did the boy go alone?" or "Was it raining when the boy and girl went for a walk?"

If the patient is not aphasic, screen for alexia by having the patient read a paragraph from a newspaper or magazine.

The examiner should note any syllable or word substitutions (paralexic errors), omitted words, and defects in comprehension.

This method of assessing reading comprehension is easily performed at the bedside; the examiner merely has to write examples of words, phrases, and sentences on a plain writing tablet. Occasionally, patients have visual field defects or problems in ocular motility. In such cases, the examiner must assist the patient in staying on the written line and ensuring that he completes one line before starting another. By careful observation and examination, the examiner can readily separate the true alexias from these problems in the mechanics of reading.

Writing

Writing must be tested in the same careful way as was reading. If the patient has evidence of aphasia, he will undoubtedly have an agraphia. Accordingly, in the aphasic patient, testing should start at the simplest level. First, have the patient write letters and numbers to dictation. Next, ask the patient to write the names of common objects or body parts. Thirdly, if the patient can successfully write single words, ask him to write a short sentence describing the weather, his job, or a picture from a magazine. Asking the patient to write his name is not always useful as name writing may be presevered even in the presence of gross agraphia. In the literate nonaphasic patient, the exam can begin with this sentence writing task. Writing to dictation is a somewhat different task that can also be tested if time allows. The aphasic patient who is unable to write spontaneously may show residual writing ability when asked to write to dictation.

Agraphia is diagnosed when basic language errors, gross spelling errors, or paragraphias (word or syllable substitutions) are present.

Writing can often show a malalignment in which the written line slants upward. This malalignment is an error in the mechanics of writing, but is not a agraphia per se.

Spelling

Spelling is a complex, little studied higher language function which is strongly associated with educational experience. For practical purposes spelling can be evaluated by asking the patient first to spell dictated words aloud and then to write them. In this way, both oral and written spelling are quickly tested. Gross errors in spelling can be detected in bedside testing; if it is important to establish an actual level of competence, standardized achievement tests must be used (see Appendix 1).

CLINICAL IMPLICATIONS

Cerebral Dominance

Approximately 90 percent of the population is considered definitely right handed. Of this 90 percent, more than 99 percent are strongly left hemisphere dominant for language.[3] Strong dominance means that damage to that hemisphere will cause aphasia whereas damage to the opposite hemisphere will spare language functions. The left hander does not, however, show the same pattern. Approximately 40 percent of left handers tend to be right hemisphere dominant for speech, while 60 percent have a left hemisphere dominance.[3] The degree of dominance is also not as strong as is found in right handers as 80 percent of all left handers have some mixed dominance for language (language functions in both hemispheres).[9] Accordingly, damage to either hemisphere in a left handed patient will result in aphasia in 80 percent of all cases. The aphasia will be less severe than that resulting from a similar lesion in the left hemisphere in a right handed patient. Knowing the patient's dominance for language is important for localizing lesions and for deciding the risk to language of neurosurgical procedures. In cases in which documentation of hemispheric dominance for language is critical (e.g., left handed patient with a right middle cerebral artery aneurysm), an intracarotid Amytal injection at the time of angiography can often establish dominance.[14]

Aphasic Syndromes

The dissolution of language secondary to brain damage is not a unitary process; all components of language can show variable impairment. The comprehensive study of right handed aphasic patients has resulted in a generally accepted schema of cortical localization of language. The posterior language area (area 1, Fig. 5-1) is the cortical area primarily concerned with the comprehension of spoken language. This area has classically been referred to as Wernicke's area, although the exact boundaries of the region have not been agreed upon.[4] The anterior language area (area 2, Fig. 5-1) subsumes the functions of language production. Brodmann's area 44 within the anterior language area is the classic Broca's area. Traditionally, patients with damage in the posterior speech area are called receptive aphasics because of their primary difficulty in understanding spoken language. Patients with lesions in the anterior area are called expressive aphasics because of their difficulty in producing language. The problem in using the term "expressive aphasia" is that all aphasics have some type of abnormal language expression; thus, the inexperienced examiner tends to classify all aphasia as "expressive aphasia." For this reason, we prefer to use the classification system described below rather than the expressive-receptive dichotomy. This classification system follows the classic anatomic pattern, is easy for the student to understand, and is useful for the clinician in localizing lesions. Because of bilateral language representation in the left handed patient, this classification system is most useful in right handed patients with left hemisphere lesions.

It is often difficult to categorize the language of the patient with an

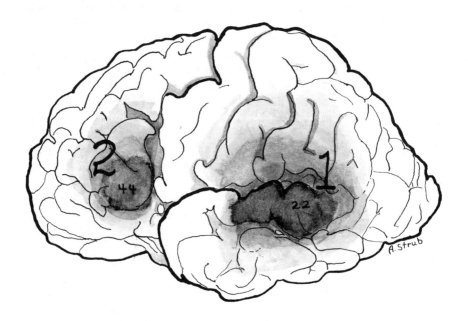

FIGURE 5-1

acute lesion. The acute destructive lesion causes maximal language disruption and is often associated with considerable disorientation and confusion. In the first few weeks, recovery is rapid and the aphasic picture constantly changes. After three weeks, the aphasic pattern is more stable and may be fully assessed. The final prognosis of language recovery is rapid and the aphasic picture constantly changes. After three weeks, the aphasic pattern is more stable and may be fully assessed. The final prognosis of language recovery, however, cannot be given at this time as the recovery process can continue for months or even years.

Global Aphasia

Global aphasia is the most common and severe form of aphasia. It is characterized by spontaneous speech that is either absent or reduced to a few stereotyped words or sounds (e.g., "ba, ba, ba" or "dis, a dis, a dis"). Performance on repetition is at the same level as spontaneous speech. Comprehension is absent or reduced to only recognition of the patient's name or a few selected words. Reading and writing are likewise obliterated. Global aphasia is caused by a large lesion that damages most or all of the combined language areas 1 and 2. The most common lesion is an occlusion of the internal carotid artery or the middle cerebral artery at its origin. Unfortunately, the prognosis is poor for language recovery in these patients. Global aphasia is almost always associated with hemiplegia. Because of these combined deficits, such patients have a severe problem in adjustment.

Broca's Aphasia

This classic syndrome has as its hallmark nonfluent, dysarthric, effortful speech. The patient utters mostly nouns and verbs (high content words) with a paucity of grammatical fillers. The characteristic speech has been called agrammatic or telegraphic. For example, one Broca's aphasic described a picture of a boy on a stool stealing cookies while his mother is washing dishes and letting the sink run over[10] in the following manner: "boy . . . ah girl steal cookie . . . . Stool falling . . . . water spilling . . . . dishes." Repetition and reading aloud are as severely impaired in these patients as is their spontaneous speech. Auditory and reading comprehension are surprisingly intact. Naming may show occasional paraphasias.

This characteristic nonfluent aphasic syndrome results from a lesion in the anterior speech area (area 2, Fig. 5-1). The lesion causing Broca's aphasia includes more than area 44 alone. Lesions restricted exclusively to area 44 result in only transient dysarthria or dysprosody.[11] Auditory and visual (reading) comprehension are intact because parietal and temporal lobes are not damaged. The Broca's aphasic usually has a right hemiplegia.

These patients often have an interesting and significant emotional change, characterized by frustration, agitation, and depression.[2] Whether this emotional change is a functional reaction to the loss of speech or a specific organic change associated with left frontal lobe damage is not yet known.

Prognosis for language recovery in Broca's aphasia is generally more favorable than in global aphasia. Because of intact comprehension, these patients adjust better to life situations.

Wernicke's Aphasia

Wernicke's aphasia can be considered the linguistic opposite of Broca's aphasia. The patient with Wernicke's aphasia has fluent, effortless, well articulated speech. The output, however, contains many paraphasias and is often devoid of substantive words. There is often a great press to speak which may overpower the listener. The following is an example of speech in Wernicke's aphasia. The patient was a ferry boat captain with a left temporal brain tumor. In describing his previous work, the patient said, "Yea, I walked on the . . . always over . . . then pull it in . . . tie the . . . ah, ah over and back over wellendy catch it . . . ."

The spontaneous speech can range from comprehensive sentences with occasional paraphasic errors to totally incomprehensible jargon in which most words are paraphasias and the output is empty and devoid of content. The essential feature of Wernicke's aphasia is a severe disturbance of auditory comprehension. Because the comprehension defect is so marked, the patients answer questions inappropriately and are unaware that their answers are often complete nonsense. Repetition is severely impaired because of the comprehension defect. Naming is grossly paraphasic. Reading and writing are also markedly impaired.

The lesion causing Wernicke's aphasia is in the posterior language area (area 1, Fig. 5-1). The more severe the defect in auditory comprehension, the more likely it is that the lesion involves the posterior portion of the superior temporal gyrus. If single word comprehension is good, yet comprehension of complex material is impaired, the lesion is more likely to involve the parietal lobe rather than the superior temporal.[10] Since the damage is restricted to parietal and temporal lobes, the classic Wernicke's aphasic does not have a hemiplegia.

The Wernicke's aphasic is often initially considered to be psychotic rather than aphasic by family and medical personnel alike. This confusion arises because the patient usually does not have a hemiplegia, and produces inappropriate, but often reasonably well formed, sentences. The gross comprehension deficit is not appreciated and the inappropriate answers to the examiner's questions are judged to be due to a basic thought disorder rather than a language disorder. The patient's brain damage is overlooked because of the absence of neurologic findings such as hemiparesis, sensory loss, or altered level of consciousness. These patients can often develop unusual behavior patterns. They are frequently totally unaware of their problem and talk endlessly without the slightest appreciation for their language deficit. This indifference may approach the point of euphoria. Other patients, however, develop a pronounced paranoid attitude with combative behavior. This behavioral change may become chronic and require major tranquilization and/or confinement to a psychiatric ward.

Patients with severe comprehension deficits do not have a good prognosis for language recovery, even with intensive speech therapy. Milder Wernicke's aphasics may evolve into conduction or anomic aphasics, conditions in which auditory comprehension is more adequate, but output contains paraphasias and word finding pauses.

Conduction Aphasia

Conduction aphasia is characterized by fluent, yet halting speech with word finding pauses and literal paraphasias. Comprehension is good, naming is mildly disturbed, but repetition is severely defective. This syndrome demonstrates that repetition and propositional speech (everyday language used to describe events or thoughts) are distinct psycholinguistic processes. In the conduction aphasic, reading is quite good, but writing shows errors in spelling, word choice, and syntax.

The lesion causing this type of aphasia is usually reported as involving the arcuate fasciculus, a long fiber tract (AF on Fig. 5-2) between the anterior and posterior areas. Thus, this entity represents one of the disconnection syndromes.[6]

Anomic Aphasia

There is a group of aphasics whose only language defects are word finding difficulty and an inability to name objects on confrontation. This condition has been labeled anomic, nominal, or amnesic aphasia. Spontaneous speech is fluent and grammatically rich, but contains word finding pauses. The patients produce paraphasias when searching for specific object names. The patient's auditory comprehension is very good, except when asked to point to a series of specific objects. This comprehension defect is a result of a two way dissociation of naming: he cannot name objects and frequently has difficulty recognizing object names when offered in examination. Repetition is good, again with the exception of sentences containing many nouns. Reading and writing

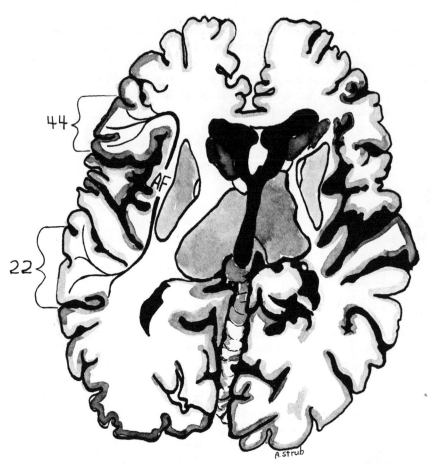

FIGURE 5-2

may or may not be impaired in specific patients; the degree of alexia and agraphia depends entirely upon the location of the lesion responsible for the aphasia.

Lesions in many parts of the dominant hemisphere can cause anomic aphasia; thus, the localizing significance of this type of aphasia is limited. The most severe anomic aphasias, however, are noted in patients with temporal lobe lesions involving the second and third temporal gyri. This area cannot be considered an actual "word dictionary" area, but includes important pathways from the occipital lobe to the limbic system that are critical for learning object names.[6] These pathways may also be important in the retrieval of previously learned names. Lesions in the parietotemporal area also result in rather severe anomia. Patients with these lesions also have substantial alexias with agraphia. Accordingly, the syndrome of alexia with agraphia and anomic aphasia will localize a lesion to the left parietotemporal area.

Anomias may be so mild that they are scarcely detectable in normal conversation, while other anomias are sufficiently severe that spontaneous output is nonfluent and empty of meaningful content. Prognosis for language recovery will be dependent upon the severity of the initial defect. Since language output is relatively spared and comprehension is reasonably intact, such patients make better life adjustments than other more severely affected aphasics.

Transcortical Aphasias

The transcortical aphasias are characterized by intact repetition of spoken language, but disruption of other language functions. Some patients will have difficulty producing language, yet have adequate comprehension; while others will produce fluent speech, yet have poor comprehension.

The patient with transcortical motor aphasia is able to repeat, comprehend, and read well, but has the restricted spontaneous speech of the Broca's aphasic. In contrast, the transcortical sensory aphasic repeats well, but does not comprehend what he hears or repeats. His spontaneous speech and naming are fluent, but paraphasic as in Wernicke's aphasia. Occasionally a patient may have a combination of transcortical motor and sensory aphasias. These patients are able to repeat long sentences, even in a foreign language, with remarkable accuracy. Repetition is very easy to initiate in these patients, even inadvertently, as they have a tendency to be echolalic (to repeat everything said within the range of their hearing).

The lesions causing transcortical aphasia are extensive crescent shaped infarcts within the borderzones between major cerebral vessels (e.g., within the frontal lobe between the territories of the anterior and middle cerebral arteries) (Fig. 5-3). Transcortical motor aphasia is seen with an anterior borderzone lesion or a high frontal lobe lesion. Transcortical sensory aphasia is caused by a posterior borderzone lesion which resembles a reversed C. These lesions spare the superior temporal and inferior frontal cortex (areas 22 and 44 and immediate environs) and the parietal perisylvian cortex. This spared perisylvian cortex is all that is required for complete and accurate language repetition. When this region is the only language area spared by combined borderzone infarcts, the resulting language deficit (echolalia) has been called an isolation syndrome.[8] The most common causes of the transcortical aphasias are: (1) anoxia secondary to decreased cerebral circulation as seen in cardiac arrest, (2) occlusion or significant stenosis of the carotid artery, and (3) anoxia due to carbon monoxide poisoning. Because of the com-

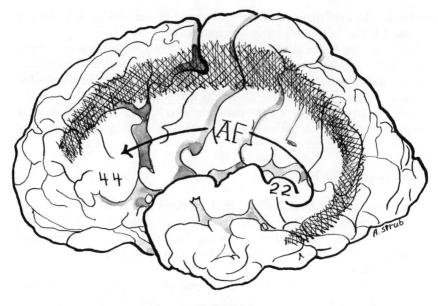

FIGURE 5-3

plex nature of these aphasias and the lack of adequate research data, prognosis as to language recovery in the transcortical aphasias is uncertain.

Pure Word Deafness

Pure word deafness is a syndrome in which patients do not have aphasic speech, agraphia, or alexia, yet have a total lack of comprehension of verbal language. Hearing is intact and auditory agnosia is not present, but the patient is "deaf" for spoken words.

The location of the lesion producing this condition is not well established, but is always in the posterior language area. A deep lesion in the temporal lobe can disconnect auditory input from the auditory cortex.

Articulation Disturbances

Pure dysarthrias are caused by lesions in any of the inputs to the muscles of articulation: the cortex as in Broca's aphasia, basal ganglia as in Parkinsonism or cerebral palsy, striatal or pontine lesions bilaterally as in pseudobulbar palsy, or the bulbar neurons as in amyotrophic lateral sclerosis. The patient with pure dysarthria will be able to communicate normally using reading and writing.

Buccofacial apraxia may be caused by various lesions between the supramarginal gyrus and the frontal lobe in the dominant hemisphere. Lesions in these areas appear to interrupt the motor planning necessary for the complex movements of normal speech. Many aphasics, particularly Broca's and conduction aphasics, have considerable apraxia of facial movement. Some patients with language output resembling Broca's aphasia may, in fact, be pure buccofacial apraxics. The difficulty in separating the aphasic and apraxic components of speech in some patients has resulted in some speech pathologists considering Broca's aphasia as merely an apraxic disorder and not a true aphasia. Broca's aphasia is seen, however, in the absence of any buccofacial apraxia. Therefore, careful examination of each patient is important to separate the apraxic and aphasic components.

Dysfluency (stuttering or stammering) is another speech production problem. This is not an aphasia, an apraxia, nor a dysarthria. It is a common speech disorder whose exact etiology is not known. Both organic and functional explanations have been advanced, but not proven.

Alexia

There are several distinct syndromes in which reading ability is impaired by acquired brain lesions. The classic syndrome of pure alexia without agraphia[5, 6] is caused by a left posterior cerebral artery occlusion in a right handed individual. The resulting cerebral infarct damages the posterior portion of the corpus callosum as well as the left occipital lobe. Since the left visual cortex is damaged, all visual information enters the right hemisphere alone. The right visual cortex perceives the written material, but is unable to transmit it to the left hemisphere because of the callosal lesion (Fig. 5-4). The inferior parietal lobule in the dominant hemisphere (primarily area 39, angular gyrus) is the association cortex that combines the visual and auditory information necessary for reading and writing. In alexia without agraphia, the inferior parietal lobule is disconnected from all visual input. Since the lobule and its connections within the language area are intact, the patient is able to write normally. One of the dramatic aspects of this syndrome is the patient's ability to write lengthy meaningful messages only to be unable to read his own writing. These patients are able to understand words spelled aloud. Interestingly, most patients with this syndrome can name objects and discuss visual events occurring in their environment. This type of visual information must cross to the left hemisphere by some pathway other than the damaged posterior corpus callosum.

A second distinct type of alexia results from damage to the inferior parietal lobule itself (angular gyrus and environs). This lesion renders the patient both unable to read and to write. This syndrome is classi-

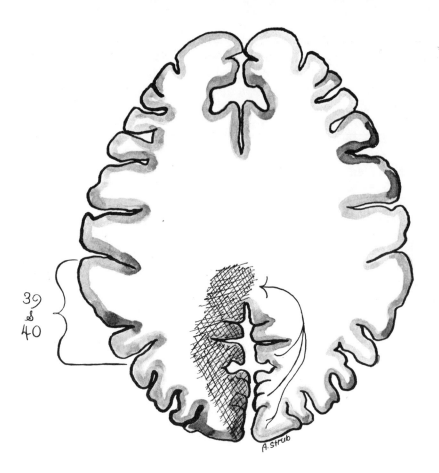

FIGURE 5-4. The cross-hatched area represents infarction of the left visual cortex and the posterior portion of the corpus callosum. The visual information from the right visual cortex (arrow) is unable to reach the left inferior parietal lobule (39 and 40) because of the callosal lesion.

cally called alexia with agraphia. These patients are not appreciably aphasic, but may have a certain degree of anomia. Recognition of this syndrome is clinically important, as in the right handed patient the lesion is invariably in the left inferior parietal area.

The most common acquired alexia is neither of the pure syndromes, but is the alexia that is associated with aphasia. In these cases comprehension of written language is impaired equally with verbal comprehension.

Agraphia

Writing is a complex motor task that involves the translation of a language item into written symbols. The linguistic message to be written originates in the posterior language area, is then translated into visual symbols in the inferior parietal area, and is finally sent to the frontal language area for motor processing. Lesions within any of these language areas will cause an agraphia. With the exception of patients with pure word deafness, all aphasics show some degree of agraphia. Although the most common agraphia is the form seen with aphasia, there are circumstances in which agraphia may be seen in the absence of aphasia. There are two agraphic syndromes seen in patients with damage in the dominant parietal lobe; the first is the agraphia seen with alexia described in the previous section, the second is a syndrome of agraphia in association with other parietal lobe signs (dyscalculia, right-left disorientation, and finger agnosia) called the Gerstmann syndrome. The Gerstmann syndrome will be discussed in detail in Chapter 9.

There is a rare pure agraphia which occurs only with the left hand. This syndrome is seen in patients with lesions of the anterior corpus callosum. These patients are agraphic with the left hand only because the right motor cortex is disconnected from the language areas of the left hemisphere. Writing with the right hand is normal because of the intact connections of the left motor cortex and the language areas. Figure 5-5 demonstrates the normal pathways required for writing. It is apparent that the callosal lesion (F_1) interrupts the language message going to the right hemisphere.

Psychotic Language

Rambling, disjointed, neologistic language can be seen in severe functional psychosis (especially schizophrenia), advanced organic dementia, and fluent jargon aphasia. Differentiation of these three conditions on the basis of their spontaneous speech alone may be difficult. Historical data are invaluable; an acute onset of gross language disturbance in the elderly favors the diagnosis of a stroke with aphasia, a prolonged history of language deterioration in the young patient favors a diagnosis of schizophrenia or an unusual organic lesion such as a left hemisphere glioma, while a gradual deterioration of language in the older patient suggests a diagnosis of dementia or other focal brain lesions such as left hemisphere tumors or subdural hematoma. Unfortunately, detailed historical information is often unavailable and a tentative diagnosis must be based upon mental status findings alone.

Each of the above conditions has certain features which help to distinguish it from the others. Systematized paranoid delusions may be seen in both aphasia and dementia. However, such delusions are more common in schizophrenia. Neologisms produced by the schizophrenic tend to be consistent and often symbolic (e.g., one paranoid schizo-

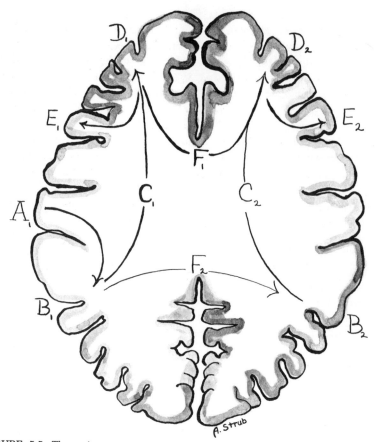

FIGURE 5-5. The written message originates in the posterior language area of the dominant hemisphere (B₁). The message is transferred via the arcuate fasciculus (C₁) to the premotor area in the same hemisphere (D₁). Motor patterns are transferred to the motor strip (E₁) for innervation of the right hand. The message must cross via the anterior corpus (F₁) to the right motor system (D₂, E₂) for innervation of the left hand. The pathway F₂. C₂ is not a significant pathway for transferring the written message to the right motor area because a lesion of the anterior callosum (F₁) is sufficient to cause agraphia of the left hand.

phrenic patient repeatedly referred to the "frinky-franks" that were placed in the walls to watch him). Neologisms produced by the aphasic tend to be random and nonsymbolic (e.g., "The walret is the you know, wimbit, lep, olla other one"). The demented patient will frequently have word finding difficulty and will produce circumlocutory speech with some neologistic paraphasias. Their speech is generally more comprehensible, however, and less paraphasic than that of the patient with aphasia.

Because it is difficult to differentiate these conditions by listening to spontaneous speech alone, complete language testing is essential. Careful comprehension testing reveals that the jargon aphasic is unable to understand even very simple commands. The demented or schizophrenic patient will have adequate comprehension, but may be difficult to evaluate because of a lack of cooperation. Testing repetition will usually demonstrate inferior performance by the aphasic. Naming tasks will clearly reveal the aphasic's language problems by his production of paraphasic errors. The aphasic shown a key may say "Pel, klo, klep, kleep . . . key," whereas the schizophrenic may call it a "key sort of watching tower thing." In this instance, the schizophrenic correctly identified the object, but incorporated it into his disordered thought process. The demented patient usually will have some naming trouble, but not as severe as that seen in aphasia nor as bizarre as seen in schizophrenia. Asked to name a key, the demented patient might well answer, "lock, no . . . one of the things you use to . . . not the lock, . . . the lock keyer, . . . key!"

The differential diagnosis of these conditions is important as a misdiagnosis may lead to gross mismanagement. For example, a very robust eighty-year-old retired grocer began answering questions inappropriately at dinner one evening. Becoming concerned, the wife continued to ask questions which the husband was unable to answer appropriately. He became frustrated, angry, and agitated. The wife became frightened and called the police. Because of his aggressive behavior, the man was jailed for three days. He was then transferred to a psychiatric hospital where he remained for an additional three days before a neurologist diagnosed a Wernicke's aphasia secondary to a middle cerebral artery thrombosis. In many cases, mistakes in the important differential diagnosis will be made unless a careful mental status examination is carried out.

Differentiating the demented from the schizophrenic patient is a more difficult task. On complete examination, the demented patient may show problems with praxis and drawing that help make the the clinical diagnosis. The demented patient may show distinct organic patterns of errors on drawings (Chap. 6). The schizophrenic often distorts drawings, but usually can make recognizable copies of designs and figures. Ideational apraxia (Chap. 9) demonstrated by asking the patient to fold a letter and place it in an envelope, is often present in the demented patient, but not in the schizophrenic. Some clues to the differential diagnosis may be obtained from the beside mental status examination, while a complete neuropsychological evaluation and other neurodiagnostic tests are often needed to make a final diagnosis.

Nonorganic Speech and Language Disorders

There are several types of functional speech disorders that can be mistaken for organic language patterns. Some neurotic patients will convert anxiety into a halting, effortful, telegraphic speech pattern (e.g., "Me want go home see wife"). These patients have normal comprehension, repetition, and naming. Reading and writing are also intact, but are carried out in the same slow effortful fashion. Mild dysarthria may also be present. These patients may require the help of both psychiatrists and speech pathologists to alter their speech patterns.

Other functional patients develop an acute aphonia (total inability to adduct the vocal cords and make audible sounds). Aphonia may arise as a pure conversion symptom or more commonly as sequela to some insult to the speech apparatus. One middle aged patient remained aphonic for two months, after awaking from surgery with an endotracheal tube in place. These patients breath normally and show no evidence of stridor. They communicate well with gesture, a mouthing of words, and writing. This type of functional overlay is well known to speech pathologists and responds well to therapy.

Elective mutism is another functional speech disorder which may be seen in either children or emotionally disturbed adults. It is characterized by a willful reluctance or an outright refusal to speak. The disorder may be complete (i.e., an absolute lack of speech in all situations) or relative (i.e., selective communication with a small circle of intimates). The speech when present may be limited to a mouthing of words, whispering, or a slow, labored, halting production. The electively mute patient typically has no language deficit and is physiologically capable of producing speech sounds. Some patients do have a basic organic language disorder with considerable emotional overlay. The mutism is often resistant to the usual forms of speech and psychotherapy,[13] but does respond to behavior modification.[12]

SUMMARY

Language is a very complex and interesting higher cognitive function. Because of the unique relationship of language and cerebral dominance, most acquired disorders of language are pathognomonic of left hemisphere damage. Careful evaluation of language functions can also localize the lesion within the dominant hemisphere. Language is of critical importance for many other cognitive functions, thus the subsequent parts of the mental status examination must be administered and interpreted with some caution in the aphasic patient.

REFERENCES

1. Benson, F.: Fluency in aphasia: Correlation with radioactive scan localization. Cortex 3:373, 1967.
2. Benson, F.: Psychiatric aspects of aphasia. Br. J. Psychiat. 123:555, 1973.

3. Benson, F., and Geschwind, N.: Cerebral dominance and its disturbances. Pediatr. Clin. N. Am. 15:759, 1968.
4. Bogan, J.: Wernicke's area—where is it? Thoughts about (and against) cortical localization. Paper presented at the 13th Annual Meeting of the Academy of Aphasia, October 5, 1975, Victoria, British Columbia.
5. Dejerine, J.: Des differentes verietes de cecite verbale. Mem. Soc. Biolog. 1892, pp. 1-30.
6. Geschwind, N.: Disconnection syndromes in animals and man. Part II. Brain 88:585, 1965.
7. Geschwind, N.: Current concepts in aphasia. N. Engl. J. Med. 284:654, 1971.
8. Geschwind, N., Quadfasel, F., and Segarra, J.: Isolation of the speech area. Neuropsychologia 6:327, 1968.
9. Gloning, I., Gloning, K., Haub, G., and Quatember, R.: Comparison of verbal behavior in right-handed and non-right handed patients with anatomically verified lesions of one hemisphere. Cortex 5:43, 1969.
10. Goodglass, H., and Kaplan, E.: The Assessment of Aphasia and Related Disorders. Lea and Febiger, Philadelphia, 1972.
11. Mohr, J., Funkenstein, H., Finkelstein, S., Pessin, M., Duncan, G., and Davis K.: Broca's area infarction versus Broca's aphasia. Paper presented at the 27th Annual Meeting of the American Academy of Neurology, April 28-May 3, 1975, Bal Harbor, Florida.
12. Norman, A., and Broman, H.: Volume feedback and generalization techniques in shaping speech of an electively mute boy: A case study. Percept. Mot. Skills 31:463, 1970.
13. Reed, G.: Elective mutism in children: A re-appraisal. J. Child Psychol. Psychiatry 4:99, 1963.
14. Wada, J.: A new method for the determination of the side of cerebral speech dominance: A preliminary report on the intercarotid injection of sodium amytal in man. Med. Biol. 14:221, 1949.

CHAPTER 6

Memory

Disturbances in memory are the most common initial complaint and often the most disabling feature of early organic brain disease. Careful attention to memory testing can often demonstrate the presence of a genuine organic disorder, even before abnormal findings are noted on standard neurologic examination. Almost all patients with presenile and senile dementia show early memory problems such as losing track of the date, forgetting work details, or failing to remember events or commitments that fall outside their daily routine. This partial amnesia is insideous and makes it impossible for the patient to function effectively. There can be devastating effects on social and vocational adjustment before the organic nature of the problem is fully appreciated. Recognition of this memory difficulty allows the clinician and the family to help the patient avoid potential personal catastrophe (e.g., the judge who is unable to remember the details of an important case in his court).

Various organic diseases result in different types of memory disturbance (e.g., severe memory deficit in relative isolation in Korsakoff's syndrome, memory difficulty compounded by inattention and agitation in the confusional states, or impaired memory associated with general cognitive dysfunction in dementia). In each of these diseases, memory is disturbed by different pathophysiologic mechanisms. Memory studies have demonstrated that there are various steps in the memory process and that each step may be localized in separate areas of the brain. These recent discoveries allow the clinician to make clinical-anatomic correlations based upon the results of careful memory testing.

Not all memory difficulties are organic in origin. Depressed patients often have apparent difficulty with their memory and may be erroneously diagnosed as having an early dementia. Since performance on memory testing requires maximum patient cooperation and effort, the depressed patient with psychomotor retardation will often perform poorly. The misdiagnosis of depression as dementia or the reverse is a serious diagnostic error that can lead to months or even years of inappropriate treatment. This is a difficult differential diagnostic problem. However, full neurologic, psychiatric, and psychologic evaluation can almost always lead to the appropriate diagnosis.

TERMINOLOGY

Memory is a general term for a mental process that allows the individual to store experiences and perceptions for recall at a later time. The time span for recall can be as short as a few seconds as in a digit repetition task or as long as many years as in the recall of childhood experiences. The memory process consists of several steps. In the first step, registration or reception, the information is registered by a particular sensory modality (e.g., touch, auditory, or visual). Once the sensory imput has been received and registered, that information is held temporarily in short term memory. The second step, retention or storage, consists of storing the information in a more permanent form (long term memory). This storage process is enhanced by repetition or by association with other information already in storage. Storage is an active process that requires considerable effort through practice and rehearsal.[13] The final step in the memory process is the recall or retrieval of the stored information. The retrieval step is an active process of mobilizing stored information. Each step in the total memory process relies upon the integrity of the previous steps. Any interruption in the hierarchy will prevent the storage or retrieval of a memory. Studies on memory have demonstrated that these memory steps have distinct neuroanatomic substrates and are subject to specific disease processes. Since different diseases can effect different aspects of memory, it is imperative that the clinician be able to separate the steps of the memory process by means of his examination.

Clinically, memory is subdivided into three basic types based upon the time span between stimulus presentation and memory retrieval. The terms "immediate," "recent," and "remote" are commonly used to denote these basic types. Unfortunately, these terms are descriptive and the time span implied is not well defined in clinical use. Immediate memory or immediate recall refers to the recall of a memory trace after an interval of a few seconds as in repetition of a series of digits. Short term memory is also used by some to describe the same task. Recent memory is a vague term that refers to the patient's capacity to remember day to day events (e.g., the date, his doctor's name, what he ate for breakfast, or recent news events). In fact, recent memory is the ability to learn new material and to retrieve that material after an interval of minutes, hours, or days. It is this lack of specificity of the time interval which makes the use of the term recent memory vague and difficult to apply clinically.

Remote memory is traditionally used to refer to very early recollections such as the names of teachers and old school friends, birth dates, and historical facts from the patient's earlier years. The same problem of vagueness discussed in the section on recent memory also applies to the term remote memory. In patients with a specific defect in new learning (recent memory), remote memory refers to the recall of events which occurred prior to the onset of the recent memory defect.

Amnesia is a general term for a defect in memory. Although the term may be applied to a broad spectrum of memory defects, it is most commonly used to label patients with severe and relatively isolated memory deficits (e.g., Korsakoff's syndrome or post-traumatic amnesia). The inability to learn new material is called anterograde amnesia, while the inability to recall events from the recent past is known as retrograde amnesia. The term amnesia is also used to refer to a hysterical neurosis of dissociative type in which the patient blocks out a period of time from his consciousness. These patients do not demonstrate a memory deficit on specific memory testing during this period.

EVALUATION

In the thorough mental status examination, the various aspects of memory must be assessed in some detail. This will allow the examiner to distinguish the type of memory deficit (if any), the degree of memory loss, and the impact of the memory deficit upon the patient's ability to function in a vocational or social role. The patient will commonly show different levels of performance on various memory tests depending upon the nature of his disorder (e.g., the Korsakoff patient will be able to respond very adequately to questions regarding more remote events, but will be totally unable to learn new material). The use of several different memory tests is also of clinical importance. Brain damaged patients will demonstrate differences in the incidence, nature, and degree of memory deficits based upon the type of test utilized and the nature and location of their lesions.[2,3,7,10]

The accurate assessment of memory requires that any question asked by the examiner be verifiable from a source other than the patient. For example, it does very little good to ask the patient when he graduated from high school or what he ate for lunch if the examiner is unable to ascertain the accuracy of the patient's response. Many patients with readily demonstrable memory deficits will deny their problem and produce confabulated answers. Such answers may appear perfectly appropriate to the naive examiner who is unable to verify the accuracy of the response. Personal information concerning the patient's social history, lifestyle, vocation, and so forth may be verified by the doctor if he has followed the patient for some time. In other cases, the patient's family can verify this information which may then be used to evaluate the patient's recall. Material which cannot be accurately verified should not be used in the assessment of memory.

Historical facts (e.g., "When was World War II?" or "Who was the president before Mr. Ford?") are commonly used by examiners to screen memory. The basic knowledge of and accordingly the ability to recall such information are closely related to the patient's basic premorbid intellectual level, education, and general social exposure. These factors must be carefully considered when using historical facts to test memory. If used at all, questions related to historical material must be tailored to the background of the individual patient and his responses must be interpreted in the context of this background information.

One of the most sensitive and valid tests of memory is to require the patient to learn new material over time. The use of such techniques eliminates some of the dangers of unverified material and unknown social background. New learning is a more active memory process that requires more expenditure of effort on the patient's part than does the mere recall of personal or historical facts.

When evaluating memory, the examiner must be aware of a number of more basic processes which can result in impaired performance, even in the patient without a true memory deficit. Performance on memory tests requires sustained attention. Accordingly, patients with disorders of attention of any etiology will be unable to perform optimally on such tests. Similarly, the patient in an acute confusional state or with a severe psychogenic disturbance, neurotic or psychotic, will have impaired attention which hinders memory performance. Disturbances of basic sensory, motor, or language systems which interfere with comprehension or expression will result in impaired memory test performance. Poor memory performance by deaf, aphasic, acutely confused, psychotic, or grossly inattentive patients reflects defects in these more basic processes and should not be misinterpreted as evidence of specific memory deficits. Valid memory testing presumes that the patient is reasonably attentive, capable of relating to and cooperating with the examiner, and has no defect impairing the comprehension or expression of language.

Because of the clinical and social importance of memory, we have selected a number of memory tests which enable the examiner to assess a variety of memory processes.

Immediate Recall (Short Term Memory)

Immediate recall is usually tested by the digit repetition task. This has been covered in detail in Chapter 4 and will not be repeated here.

Orientation

The patient's ability to orient himself with respect to person (who he is), time (the date, etc.), and place (where he is) is important preliminary information and should be evaluated early in the examination of memory functioning.

Directions. The patient should be asked the following questions in sequence. Questions may be paraphrased when necessary to ensure clarity.

1. Person
   a. Name   What is your name?
   b. Age   How old are you?
   c. Birthdate   When was your birthday?
                                     (day, month, year)

2. Place
   a. Location   Where are we right now?
                                     What is the name of this place?
                                     What kind of place are we in now?
   b. Address   What is your home address?
   c. City location   What city are we in now?
3. Time
   a. Date   What is today's date?
                                     (year, month, date)
   b. Day of the week   What is the day, today?
                                     What day of the week is it?
   c. Time of the day   What time is it right now?
   d. Season of the year   What season is it now?
   e. Time duration   How long have you been in the
                                     hospital?
                                     How long have we been talking?

Remote Memory

Tests in this section evaluate the patient's ability to recall events of both a personal and historical nature from his store of memories. As emphasized, personal events must be verifiable by a reliable source other than the patient; the performance on the recall of historical information must be interpreted in the light of the patient's premorbid intelligence, education, and social experience.

1. Personal information
   a. Where were you born?
   b. School information: Where did you go to grade (high) school?
                                     When did you attend grade (high) school?
                                     Where is your grade (high) school located?

c. Vocational history: What do you do for work?
                              Where have you worked?
                              When did you work at those places?
d. Family information: What is your wife's (children's) name?
                              How old is your wife (children)?
                              What was your mother's maiden name?

2. Historical facts
   a. Ask the patient to name four presidents since 1900. The normal
      patient should be able to accomplish this task without difficulty.
   b. Ask the patient to name the last war in which the United States
      was directly involved. At the time of this writing, the correct re-
      sponse would be the war in Viet Nam; appropriate changes must
      be made if events supercede this.

New Learning Ability

This section assesses the patient's ability to actively learn new material
(to lay down new memories). Adequate performance requires the integrity of the total memory system: recognition and registration of the initial
sensory input, retention and storage of the information, and recall or retrieval of the stored information. An interruption in any of these stages
will impair new learning ability. A careful clinical examination of how
the patient fails a particular task may often provide valuable information
as to the nature of the impaired process.

Four Unrelated Words

Directions. Tell the patient, "I am going to tell you four words that
I would like you to remember. In a few minutes, I will ask you to recall
these words." Ensure that the patient has heard, understood, and initially
retained the four words, by having him repeat the words after presentation. Correct any errors he may make on immediate repetition. To
eliminate possible mental rehearsal, interference should be used between
presentation and recall of the words. Accordingly, the examiner may wish
to present the four words prior to the remote memory examination. After
five minutes, ask for the recall of the four words. Information concerning
the duration of memory can be obtained by asking for a recall of the words
after 10 and 30 minutes. The following words have been selected because
of their semantic and phonemic diversity.

Test Items.

1. Brown   3. Tulip
2. Honesty   4. Eyedropper

Scoring. The nonretarded patient is expected to accurately recall the four words after a 10 minute delay. After a 30 minute delay at least three of the four words should be recalled. Less adequate performance indicates a deficit in the ability to learn and recall new material over time. When a patient is unable to recall any of the four words, it is often possible to obtain an indication of some memory storage by the use of verbal cues. Semantic cues relating to the category of the named object (e.g., "one word was a color"), phonemic cues utilizing syllabic components of the word (e.g., "Hon … hones … honest … honesty"), and contextual cues (e.g., "A common flower in Holland is a_____") may be used. If a patient is unable to spontaneously recall words or to recall words with cues, the examiner may resort to asking him if he recognizes the appropriate word from a series (e.g., "Was the color red, green, brown, or yellow?").

Verbal Story For Immediate Recall

Directions. Tell the patient, "I am going to read you a short paragraph. Listen carefully, because when I finish reading, I want you to tell me everything that I told you. Do you understand?" After reading the story, say, "Now tell me everything that you can remember of the story. Start at the beginning of the story and tell me all that happened." The separate items in the story are indicated by slash (/) marks. As the patient retells the story, indicate the number of ideas recalled.

Test Item. William Stern / a 63-year-old / state representative / from Walton County / Utah / was planning his reelection campaign / when he began experiencing chest pain. / He entered Logan Memorial Hospital / for three days of medical tests. / A harmless virus was diagnosed / and he, his wife /Sandra, / and their two sons / Rick and Tommy / hit the campaign trail again./

Scoring. The story contains 15 relatively separate ideas or information items. In our experience, the average patient should be expected to produce at least eight of these items on immediate recall. Less adequate performance by the nonretarded patient indicates defective verbal recall ability.

Visual Memory (Hidden Objects)

Directions. Visual memory testing should be used with all patients, but is especially useful in evaluating the memory of aphasics. The examiner may utilize any four small, easily recognizable, objects which may be readily hidden in the patient's vicinity. We have commonly used items such as a pen, watch, keys, coins, eye glasses, etc. The use of four items provides a reasonable span for most patients. The objects are hidden while the patient is watching. Name each item as it is hidden to ensure that the patient is aware of what object was hidden in what area. After hiding the four objects, the examiner should provide interfering stimulation in the form of another mental status task, asking the patient routine questions, or engaging him in general conversation. An interference period of 10 minutes should suffice. After this period, ask the patient to find each of the hidden objects. If the patient is unable to recall the location of any object, ask him to name the hidden object. The location of named, unfound objects may be cued by the examiner.

Scoring. The average patient should find each of four hidden objects after a 10 minute delay without difficulty. Less adequate performance indicates impaired visual memory.

Visual Memory (Visual Design Reproduction)

Directions. The following subtest utilizes four simple line drawings of increasing complexity. We recommend that the examiner provide standardized stimuli cards to ensure uniformity, although the examiner may chose to draw each design at the bedside. The patient is required to reproduce each of the four designs on a piece of white paper after a five second presentation of the design and a five second delay before beginning. The following instructions are given: "I am now going to show you some simple drawings. I want you to look at the drawing as I show it to you. Be sure to look at it carefully so that you can draw what you have seen from memory. Do not draw the design until I have told you to begin." The examiner then holds each design in turn at right angles to the patient's line of sight. After withdrawing the design and waiting five seconds, tell the patient to draw the picture (see Fig. 6-1).

Scoring. Each design may be scored on a four point scale with values from 0 to 3. The higher the score, the more adequate the reproduction. The following scoring system may be used to aid the examiner in quantifying performance on this test:

0—Poor	Given for a failure to recall and reproduce the design.
1—Fair	Given for recognizable, but distorted, rotated, partially omitted, or confabulated designs.
2—Good	Given for easily recognizable designs with minor errors of integration, omission, or addition.
3—Excellent	Given for perfect (or near perfect) reproductions of the items with all appropriate components, placements, and integration.

Representative clinical examples of poor, fair, good, and excellent

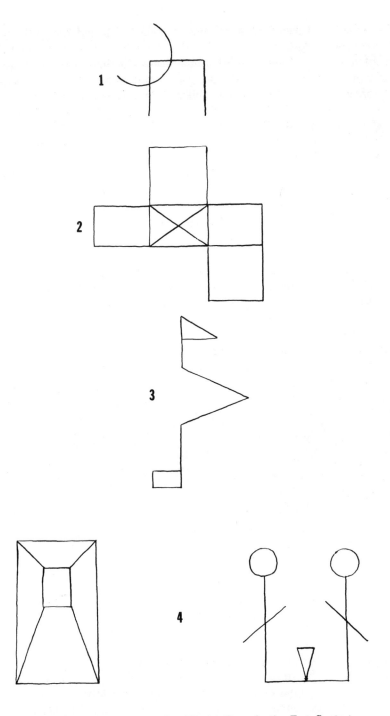

FIGURE 6-1. Test items for Visual Design Reproduction Test. See text.

drawings are shown in Figures 6-2 through 6-5 to aid the examiner in rating each design.

The average patient should produce reproductions of each design at the 2 and 3 scoring levels. All designs should be recalled. Less adequate performance indicates a deficit in visual memory.

Paired Associate Learning

Directions. Tell the patient, "I am going to read you a list of words, two at a time. Listen carefully because I will expect you to remember the words that go together. For example, if the words were big—little, I would expect you to say the word little after I said the word big." When the patient is clear as to the directions, continue as follows: "Now listen carefully to the words as I read them." Read the first presentation at the rate of one pair every two seconds. After reading the first presentation, test for recall by presenting the first recall list. Give the first word of a pair and allow five seconds for a response. If the patient gives a correct response, say, "That's right" and proceed with the next pair. If the patient gives an incorrect response, say, "No," provide the correct association, and proceed to the next pair.

After the first recall has been completed, allow a 10 second interval and give the second presentation list, proceeding as before.

Test Items.

Presentation Lists

First Presentation	Second Presentation
Weather—Bag	House—Income
High—Low	Weather—Bag
House—Income	Book—Page
Book—Page	High—Low

Recall Lists

First Recall	Second Recall
House—	High—
High—	House—
Weather—	Book—
Book—	Weather—

Scoring. The nonretarded patient is expected to recall the two "easy" paired associates (high—low, book—page) and at least one of the "hard" associates on the first recall trial, and to recall all paired associates on the second trial. Less adequate performance is indicative of impaired new learning ability. Some patients will be able to learn the paired words with strong natural associations, but are unable to learn the pairs with-

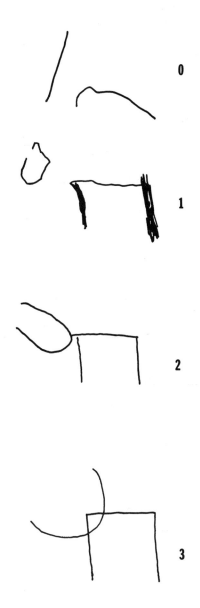

FIGURE 6-2. Renderings of design 1, Figure 6-1 with scores of 0 (poor) through 3 (excellent).

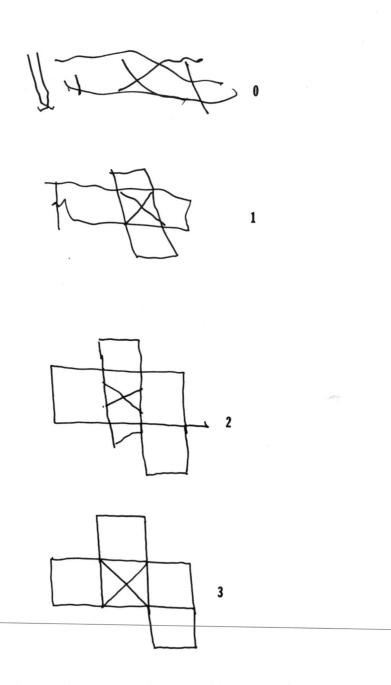

FIGURE 6-3. Renderings of design 2, Figure 6-1 with scores of 0 (poor) through 3 (excellent).

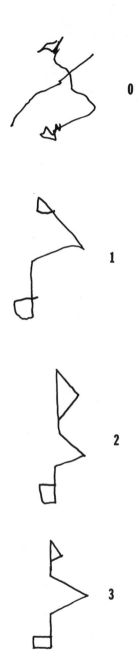

FIGURE 6-4. Renderings of design 3, Figure 6-1 with scores of 0 (poor) through 3 (excellent).

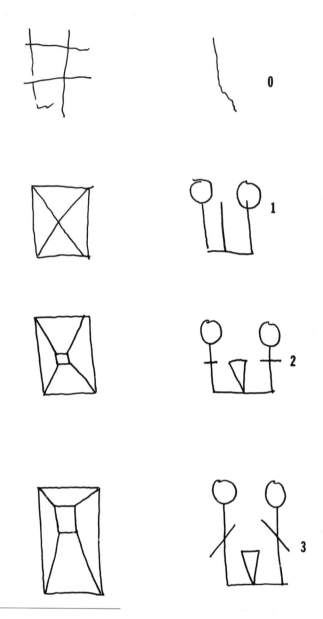

FIGURE 6-5. Renderings of design 4, Figure 6-1 with scores of 0 (poor) through 3 (excellent).

out such associations. This discrepancy demonstrates a reliance upon semantic cues and inability to learn new material which cannot be associated with memories already in storage.

CLINICAL IMPLICATIONS

Each step in the memory process requires the action of a specific neuronal system. Pathologic studies have amply documented the structures involved in the long term storage and retrieval of recent information.[5, 15, 18] The structure required for immediate recall and remote memory is not as well established pathologically. However, clinical inference does allow the prediction of the neuroanatomic substrates of these processes. Although all memories, visual, verbal, and tactile, are most likely stored in the neocortex, there are many subcortical structures necessary for the total memory process (registration, storage, and retrieval). Damage or disruption of cortical or subcortical systems will result in different patterns of dysfunction. Accordingly, the anatomy of memory is discussed in a way that allows the correlation of specific structure, memory type, and clinical condition.

Immediate Recall

The immediate recall of digits is a process that does not require any long term storage of information, but does require initial registration, short term holding, and verbal repetition. This entire process can be carried out by the language cortex surrounding the sylvian fissure. This has been demonstrated in patients with transcortical aphasia.[8] The exact mechanism by which these short term memories are maintained within the language system is not known. Reverberating circuits may be established or patterns of cortical after-image may be present. Whatever change does occur, it is not long lasting. Efficient short term memory is not a passive process. A digit sequence task will be performed much better if active mental rehearsal takes place. Digits are typically presented at one second intervals, but each digit takes approximately 200 milliseconds to present. The 800 milliseconds between digits allows ample time for rehearsal and thus increased efficiency in repetition. If the patient actively groups digits into two or three digit sets, his performance will improve. A third and always very important element in all memory processing is the association of the new material with previously stored information. A digit sequence that is similar to an old phone number or address will be much more easily recalled than a completely unique random sequence. There is usually very limited storage of information presented in this fashion. Short term memory (immediate recall) is a distinct property of the cortical sensory, motor, and integrative areas necessary to register, recall, and produce the original stimulus. It does not require the systems necessary for long term storage and permanent memory formation.

If there is any damage or disruption of these basic sensory or motor areas, then short term memory will be faulty. In digit repetition, the language system is essential, so any degree of aphasia (excluding the transcortical aphasias) can cause disruption of immediate memory functioning. This repetition failure is particularly pronounced in conduction aphasia.[17] The primary deficit in conduction aphasia is an inability to repeat. Whether this repetition failure is a defect in language or short term memory is an open question that may in fact reflect an argument of semantics.

Probably the most common cause of failure on short term memory tasks is inattention. If a patient's attention strays from the stimulus during presentation, the information will be imperfectly registered. Similarly, if the patient is inattentive during the repetition phase and time pauses occur, the memory trace will fade. Inattention can be organic as in confusional states and dementia or functional as in anxiety and depression. The clinical implications of these attentional disturbances are discussed fully in Chapters 2 and 3.

The demented patient will have difficulty with immediate memory for several reasons; such patients are often inattentive, they have cortical atrophy which affects their basic language and other sensory motor integration systems, and they have general intellectual deterioration.

There does not seem to be a distinct neuroanatomic structure for immediate memory and all patients with short term memory deficits are either inattentive, aphasic, demented, or have a specific dysfunction of the sensory system being tested (e.g., visual memory impairment in a patient with a visual perceptual disturbance secondary to a right hemisphere parieto-occipital lesion). If short term memory testing reveals specific deficits, the examiner must be very cautious when evaluating other memory processes.

Recent Memory

The ability to store and then retrieve new material (recent memory, new learning, memorizing, or long term memory) presumes intact registration, retention, and short term storage. In addition, certain specific limbic structures are required to ensure long term storage and retrieval. The hippocampi, the mamillary bodies, and the dorsal medial nuclei of the thalami are essential subcortical links in the storage and retrieval of both verbal and nonverbal memories.[15,18] The interested reader wishing further information regarding limbic anatomy is referred to any comprehensive neuroanatomy text, e.g., Crosby and coworkers.[4] Actual memories are probably not stored in these structures, but the limbic system seems to act as the mechanism to store and retrieve memories from the cortex.

Whenever these subcortical structures are destroyed or severely damaged, the patient is rendered unable to learn new material (anterograde amnesia) or to retrieve memories from the recent past (retrograde amnesia). These patients literally become fixed in time and are unable to record the passing of events from that time onward. There are certain clinical situations in which these limbic structures are damaged in isolation. Such patients develop a profound organic amnesic state. This condition is characterized clinically by the following findings: (1) severe anterograde amnesia, (2) moderate to severe retrograde amnesia, which can extend back for several years, and usually (3) confabulation in the acute stage. In the face of this devastating memory impairment, the patients have remarkably intact short term memory as assessed by digit repetition and other short term memory tests. These patients also demonstrate no change in their premorbid levels of intelligence. They carry on coherent intelligent conversations that appear abnormal only when recent events are discussed. Because the patients do not remember the date, place, and recent events, they appear confused. This confusion which is due to their memory problems can be easily misinterpreted as the classic acute confusional state described in Chapter 3. Careful observation and testing will prevent this diagnostic error.

This dramatic organic amnesic state has been seen secondary to bilateral temporal lobectomy, herpes simplex encephalitis, and bilateral hippocampal infarction. In these cases, the hippocampus has been completely destroyed bilaterally. A similar memory deficit is seen clinically in Korsakoff's syndrome (a syndrome of thiamine depletion seen in chronic alcoholism). In Korsakoff's syndrome, the lesions involve bilateral destruction to the mamillary bodies and the dorsal medial nuclei of the thalamus. The Korsakoff patient frequently goes through an acute encephalopathy (Wernicke's encephalopathy) at the onset of his memory difficulty.

In Alzheimer's dementia, patients also have defects in new learning. This defect is due to a gradual degeneration of the cells in the hippocampus. As deterioration of the hippocampal cells is the first pathologic finding in this dementia, recent memory problems are often the first clinical sign of the disease. The memory loss in the atrophic dementias is complex and will be discussed more fully in the section dealing with remote memory.

The most familiar amnesia to the layman is the memory loss that occurs after head injury. Patients with acute head injury usually have transient difficulty learning and almost always have some degree of retrograde amnesia for the time preceding the injury. In head trauma, the temporal lobes are commonly concussed against the bony confines of the middle fossa. This trauma causes a physiologic disruption of hippocampal function which in turn disturbs memory storage and retrieval. Post-traumatic amnesia is usually reversible, but in cases of significant temporal lobe damage, the memory loss can be permanent. Repeated concussion such as that seen in boxers may result in gradual, but permanent memory disturbance. An interesting feature of the amnesia seen with acute head injury is that the retrograde amnesic period will shorten in the days following recovery of consciousness. Initially the patient may not recall events occurring years preceding the accident. Within 10 days he may remember all but the few minutes immediately before the accident. This shrinking retrograde amnesia verifies that the injury did not eliminate the memories from storage, but merely rendered them temporarily irretrievable.[1]

Transient global amnesia is another curious type of organic memory problem. This syndrome probably involves transient ischemia of both medial temporal lobes secondary to decreased perfusion in the territory of the posterior cerebral arteries.[9,11] This syndrome is characterized by an acute, but temporary, confusional state with amnesia. The patients are disoriented to time and place and have a significant defect in new learning ability. Recovery generally occurs within hours or days and the patient is left with a permanent amnesia only for the duration of the episode itself. Fortunately, most episodes of transient global amnesia are temporary, although permanent memory loss has been seen in patients suffering bilateral hippocampal infarction.[6] The following case illustrates some of the essential features of this syndrome:

Dr. J. L. was a robust 68-year-old educator who was addressing a teacher's convention. In the middle of his speech he stopped suddenly, became dazed, and began to ask where he was. He repeatedly asked, "What am I doing and where am I?" On initial neurologic examination, he was distraught and very confused. He was unable to attend well and was unable to learn new material. He did not remember arriving in New Orleans, but did know that he was scheduled to attend the convention. One day later, his mental function was essentially normal except that he was amnesic for the day prior to and the day of his amnesic episode.

All of the conditions discussed thus far have resulted from bilateral lesions localized in limbic structures. While it is true that a bilateral lesion is necessary to produce a profound memory loss, there is some loss of specific memory functions following unilateral lesions. Unilateral dominant temporal lobectomy patients show a relative decrease in verbal learning, whereas patients with unilateral nondominant temporal lobectomies demonstrate a decrease in visual memory.[12]

There are various factors other than specific limbic damage that can interfere with the storage and retrieval of new material; some of these have been discussed in the previous section, but they merit additional mention here. Inattention will prevent any patient from accurately storing new material. Efficient memory storage requires close attention to the information for short term registration and continued attention and rehearsal for storage. For this reason, new learning cannot be validly tested in the inattentive patient. The aphasic is also at a tremendous disadvantage in any verbal learning task; if he cannot accurately comprehend or repeat verbal material, it is not valid to judge his memory capacity using that material. Nonverbal memory tasks are necessary to validly assess memory in the aphasic patient. Memory test performance and intelligence are directly related, accordingly the patient's premorbid intellectual level must be considered in interpreting the results of memory testing. Deficits in basic sensory capacity (i.e., hearing and vision) are sometimes overlooked in testing, but obviously sensory systems must be adequate for memory testing in each specific modality.

The patient's emotional state can also significantly effect new learning ability. The very anxious patient will make errors due to inattention and distractability. The depressed patient performs poorly on memory testing because of his inability to put forth the required effort to memorize the presented material. Poor performance on memory tests is probably the single most important factor resulting in the misdiagnosis of depression as dementia.[14] Accordingly, in the patient with psychomotor retardation and memory problems, the diagnosis of depression must be considered and pursued in the evaluation process.

Remote Memory

When a memory has remained in a person's repertoire for a number of years, it can be considered a remote or old memory. These memories are stored in the appropriate association cortex (e.g., language cortex for words or names). In contrast to recent memory, remote memory does not require the limbic system for retrieval from storage. Patients with Korsakoff's syndrome or bilateral temporal lobectomy can accurately discuss personal and historical events that occurred 10 years previously (remote memory), yet are unable to remember what they had for breakfast that morning (recent memory).[16] There is apparently a mechanism, thusfar unexplained, by which memories finally become sufficiently well established that they can be recalled without the aid of subcortical limbic structures. These remote memories can be lost only by damage to the cortical storage areas themselves. This loss of remote or old memories is seen in patients with the atrophic dementias (Alzheimer's, Pick's, and senile) or with any disease that damages extensive areas of the cortex. The memory disturbance in the demented patient is complex; such patients have difficulty with short term memory because of atrophy in the basic sensory association cortex (e.g., language cortex for verbal memory), they are hampered in recent memory acquisition because of degeneration of cells in the hippocampal system, and they have defects in remote memory because of widespread cortical atrophy.

Functional Memory Disturbances

Not all memory disorders are of organic origin and knowledge of the functional disturbances of memory is important. The interference with memory performance that can occur secondary to anxiety and depression has been discussed previously. There are, however, several psychiatric conditions in which memory disturbances are central features. The first and most common is the dissociative state seen in hysterical neurosis. This is the classic amnesic spell which has been popularized in the lay press. The patient either loses the memory of his identity completely and is unable to remember who he is or where he is (fugue state) or has periods of minutes, hours, or days when he carries out his normal life routine, but will suddenly be aware that he remembers nothing of what transpired during this period (dissociative state). During a dissociative or fugue state, the patient does not act confused like the person with transient global amnesia and is able to learn new material unlike patients with organic amnesia. There should be no difficulty differentiating the organic amnesic who cannot learn new material when tested from the hysterical amnesic who has experienced a "memory lapse." Brief testing with the four unrelated words task or paired associate words should suffice.

There is one other curious pseudomemory disturbance, the Ganser syndrome or the syndrome of approximate answers. This pseudodementia is occasionally seen in prisoners or psychiatric inpatients, many of whom have a history of previous head trauma. These patients will routinely give approximate answers to all questions, e.g., today is Tuesday (actually Wednesday), the month is March (actually April), or 2 and 2 are 5. This is an uncommon syndrome, but one that should be recognized as a pseudodementia and not a true amnesia or dementia. The functional nature of the Ganser syndrome may be readily determined by the consistently inconsistent nature of the patient's responses to any question asked.

SUMMARY

In general, memory is a hierarchical process in which information must first be registered in a basic sensory cortical area and then processed through the limbic system for new learning to occur. Finally, the material is permanently established in the appropriate association cortex. At this point, limbic retrieval is no longer required in the recall process. The immediate recall system is disturbed by damage to the primary sensory or motor cortex or by inattention. Learning is prevented by damage to the hippocampi or the mamillary bodies/medial thalamic nuclei. Old remote memories are resistant to limbic damage, but will be lost when widespread cortical damage occurs. Careful testing of the various aspects of memory can frequently lead to both a clinical and an anatomic diagnosis.

REFERENCES

1. Benson, D., and Geschwind, N.: Shrinking retrograde amnesia. J. Neurol. Neurosurg. Psychiatry 30:539, 1967.
2. Benton, A., and Spreen, O.: Visual memory test performance in mentally deficient and brain-damage patients. Am. J. Ment. Defic. 68:630, 1964.
3. Bisiach, E., and Faglioni, P.: Recognition of random shapes by patients with unilateral lesions as a function of complexity, association value, and delay. Cortex 10:101, 1974.
4. Crobsy, E., Humphrey, T., and Lauer, E.: Correlative Anatomy of the Nervous System. MacMillan, New York, 1962.
5. DeJong, R., Itabashi, H., and Olson, J.: Memory loss due to hippocampal lesions. Arch. Neurol. 20:339, 1969.
6. DeJong, R.: The hippocampus and its role in memory. J. Neurol. Sci. 19:73, 1973.
7. DeRenzi, E.: Nonverbal memory and hemispheric side of lesion. Neuropsychologia 6:181, 1968.
8. Geschwind, N., Quadfasel, F., and Segarra, J.: Isolation of the speech area. Neuropsychologia 6:327, 1968.
9. Heathfield, K., Croft, P., and Swash, M.: The syndrome of transient global amnesia brain 96:729, 1973.
10. Lewinsohn, P., Zieler, R., Libet, J., Eyeberg, S., and Nielson, G.: A comparison between frontal and nonfrontal right and left hemisphere brain-damaged patients. J. Comp. Physiol. Psychol. 81:248, 1972.
11. Mathew, N., and Meyer, J.: Pathogenesis and natural history of transient global amnesia. Stroke 5:303, 1974.
12. Milner, B.: Intellectual functions of the temporal lobes. Psychol. Bull. 51:42, 1954.
13. Neisser, U.: Cognitive Psychology. Appleton-Century-Crofts, New York, 1967.
14. Nott, P., and Fleminger, J.: Presenile dementia: the difficulties of early diagnosis. Acta Psychiat. Scand. 51:210, 1975.
15. Scoville, W., and Milner, B.: Loss of recent memory after bilateral hippocampal lesions. J. Neurol. Neurosurg. Psychiatry 20:11, 1957.
16. Selzer, B., and Benson, F.: The temporal pattern of retrograde amnesia in Korsakoff's disease. Neurology 24:527, 1974.
17. Strub, R., and Gardner, H.: The repetition defect in conduction aphasia: Mnestic or linguistic? Brain Language 1:241, 1975.
18. Victor, M., Adams, R., and Collins, G.: The Wernicke-Korsakoff Syndrome. F. A. Davis, Philadelphia, 1971.

CHAPTER 7

Constructional Ability

Constructional tasks such as line drawings, block designs, and match stick constructions are extremely useful in detecting organic brain disease and should be included in all mental status examinations. Constructional ability (constructional praxis) can be defined as the capacity to draw or construct two or three dimensional figures or shapes from one and two dimensional units. Copying line drawings with pencil on paper, reproducing match stick patterns, and reconstructing block designs are all examples of routinely employed tests of constructional ability. This high level nonverbal cognitive function is very complex and involves an integration of occipital, parietal, and frontal lobe function. Because of the extensive cortical area necessary to perform constructional tasks, early brain damage frequently disrupts performance. In some patients the unsuccessful attempt to copy a simple line drawing can be the only objective evidence suggesting organic brain disease.

Despite their importance and proven clinical utility, constructional tasks are frequently not included in bedside or office mental status testing. This is due in part to the fact that very few patients will actually complain of constructional impairment. Architects or engineers whose profession require such abilities might notice difficulties when drawing plans, reading blueprints, or translating plans into actual construction. Most patients, however, are quite surprised to find that they are unable to draw a clock or copy a block design when asked to do so. Since constructional tests take only a few minutes to perform and can yield very valuable data, we encourage every clinician to use them when performing routine mental status testing.

The term constructional ability rather than the more classic term constructional praxis will be used to discuss this general area of cognitive function. Praxis, in the strict sense, refers to the motor integration employed in the execution of complex learned movements. The reproduction of line drawings or block designs involves more than the organization of skilled hand movements. Such reproduction requires accurate visual perception, integration of perception into kinesthetic images, and translation of kinesthetic images into the final motor patterns necessary to produce the construction. The patient does not have to recognize or name the figure, but only develop an accurate concept or gestalt. The relationship of angles and sides, orientation on the page, and three dimensionality must all be appreciated if accurate motor integration is to be carried out. The final step, of course, requires adequate limb strength and coordination.

Constructional impairment rather than constructional apraxia will be used to describe the failure to perform adequately on any of these various tasks. As implied in the preceding paragraph, a disturbance in praxis (apraxia) is merely a breakdown in the execution of the learned movements involved in the constructional task.[7] The term apraxia excludes the component of visual perception and thus does not accurately describe the neuropsychologic complexity of the process. It is true that pure limb apraxia (Chap. 9) can cause failure but so can faulty visual perception, spatial orientation, or right-left sense. For this reason, the more inclusive term constructional impairment will be used.

EVALUATION

As we have mentioned, constructional ability may be tested in a variety of ways. Different levels of performance can often be found in the same patient on the different tests. As an example of the range of test materials which may be employed, Warrington[16] has listed the following six basic types of tests which can be used to elicit evidence of constructional impairment: (1) two dimensional block designs, (2) paper and pencil reproduction of geometric shapes, (3) spontaneous drawings, (4) stick pattern reproduction, (5) three dimensional block constructions, and (6) spatial analysis tasks requiring the patient to shade in the portion of a design which is common to two or more overlapping figures. Patients with brain lesions do show differences in the incidence, severity, and quality of constructional impairment depending upon the type of test used and the nature and location of their lesions.[1,3,13]

The clinical examination of constructional impairment in the individual patient should ideally include several tests to tap somewhat different aspects of constructional ability. Drawings to command and reproduction drawings remain the most easily administered and interpreted tests and are strongly recommended as essential elements of the routine mental status examination.

The use of the tests outlined in this book presumes that the patient has adequate vision (20/100 as objectively tested) and sufficient motoric ability to effectively use paper, pencil, and blocks. Deficits in either motor or sensory channels will hinder performance. Impairment secondary to these problems does not reflect a disruption in the higher cortical function these tests are designed to assess. A number of constructional tests which include a memory component are available.[4,8,12] While the inclusion of the memory component does increase the sensitivity of constructional tests of brain dysfunction, it also raises serious problems in the interpretation of the test results. Deficits in drawings from memory may be due to memory or constructional problems or a combination of the two. We feel that memory is a sufficiently important variable that it should be specifically tested in isolation. As we have stressed throughout this examination, a primary goal of each aspect of mental status testing is to assess as discrete a cognitive function as possible. Accordingly, no memory for designs tests are included in this handbook. The reader is referred to the appendix for further information regarding the availability and description of these tests.

The following brief tests of constructional ability have been included for bedside and office testing. These tests have been chosen because of their ease of administration and interpretation, a limited need for apparatus and specialized equipment, and their proven efficacy in the detection of diffuse and focal brain lesions.

Reproduction Drawings

Directions. We suggest that reproduction drawings be administered first when assessing constructional ability because of their apparent simplicity and familiarity. The drawings presented below are organized in order of increasing difficulty and should be administered in this order for all patients. Both two and three dimensional drawings are used because of frequent quantitative and qualitative performance differences noted on these two somewhat different tasks. The examiner may either use a standard predrawn set of designs (probably best because the stimuli are identical for each administration and generally of better quality than quickly drawn bedside examples) or draw the stimulus figures on the left side of a piece of blank white paper for each administration. The use of separate sheets of paper for each design is advised for patients who are highly distractable or perseverative. The use of lined progress note forms, consult sheets, and other handy, but perceptually confusing, paper is not recommended. It is often useful to use two colors of pencil or felt tip pen to reduce the possibility of confusion between the drawings of the patient and those drawn by a hurried examiner. Each design should be administered to every patient despite obvious constructional impairment on early drawings. Patients' frustrations with their efforts may be reduced by further encouragement by the examiner.

Introduce each item by saying "Please draw this design exactly as it looks to you" (see Fig. 7-1).

Scoring. To aid the examiner in quantifying the adequacy of patients performance on this test, an objective scoring system[15] is provided for rating the relative quality of each drawing.

0—Poor   Given for nonrecognizable reproductions or a gross distortion of the basic design gestalt.

1—Fair   Given for moderately distorted or rotated two dimen-

Horizontal Diamond

Two Dimensional Cross

Three Dimensional Cube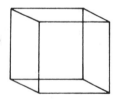

Three Dimensional Pipe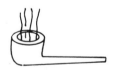

FIGURE 7-1. Test items for Reproduction Drawings Test. See text.

sional drawings or a loss of all three dimensionality with moderate distortions or rotations on three dimensional designs.

2—Good   Given for minimal distortion or rotations with adequate integration on two dimensional designs and some evidence of three dimensionality, but less than perfect reproduction on three dimensional designs.

3—Excellent   Given for perfect (or near perfect) reproductions of two and three dimensional drawings.

Patients' drawings showing evidence of rotations of more than 90 degrees (see Fig. 7-2, example 1), perseveration (see Fig. 7-2, example 2), or "closing in" (see Fig. 7-2, example 3) are given ratings of 0.

Although the physician will soon gain familiarity with this test and develop his own scoring criteria based upon experience, examples from our clinical population of poor, fair, good, and excellent drawing reproductions are shown in Figures 7-3 to 7-6 to aid the examiner in rating each design.

Drawings To Command

Directions. The three drawings in Figure 7-7 were selected from those commonly used by neurologists in the clinical examination of patients. They are a representative sample which can readily assess auditory-motor transposition, visual neglect, and constructional ability. The patient is required to draw each of the following pictures to verbal command on a blank piece of white paper. Introduce the test by saying "I would now like you to draw some simple pictures on this paper. Draw each picture as well as you are able. Please draw a picture of a clock with the numbers and hands on it; a daisy in a flower pot; a house in perspective so that you can see two sides and the roof."

Scoring. A simple scoring system similar to that used with reproduction drawings may be used to aid the examiner in quantifying performance on this test.

0—Poor   Given for nonrecognizable drawings or a gross distortion of the basic gestalt.

1—Fair   Given for moderate distortion or rotation of any of the drawings or a loss of three dimensionality on the house drawing. The clock should contain one of the following: an approximately circular face or the numbers 1 through 12. The daisy should be recognizable as a flower in a pot and the house recognizable as a house.

2—Good   Given for only mild distortions with adequate integration on all pictures. The house should contain some

Example 1 ROTATION

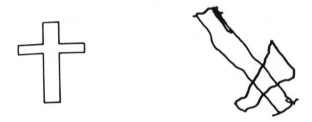

Example 2 PERSEVERATION

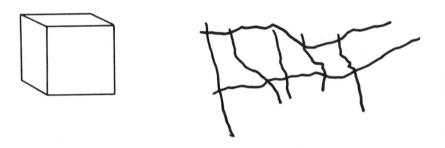

Example 3 "Closing In"

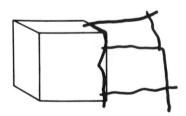

FIGURE 7-2. Examples of patient drawings with specific types of errors.

0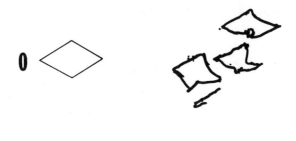

1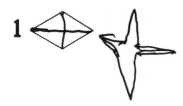

2

3

FIGURE 7-3. Renderings of Horizontal Diamond Test with scores of 0 (poor) through 3 (excellent).

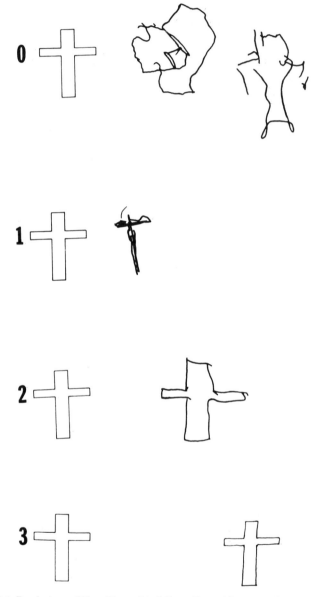

FIGURE 7-4. Renderings of Two Dimensional Cross Test with scores of 0 (poor) through 3 (excellent).

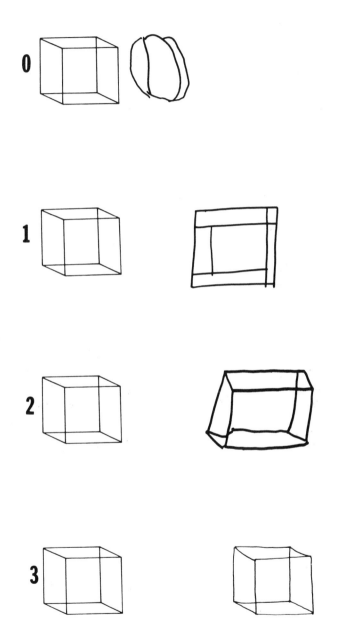

FIGURE 7-5. Renderings of Three Dimensional Cube Test with scores of 0 (poor) through 3 (excellent).

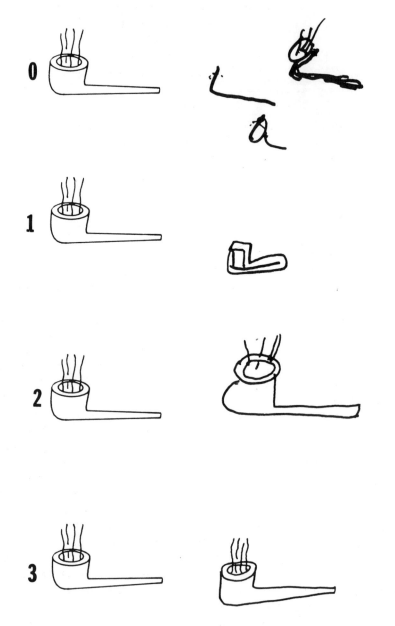

FIGURE 7-6. Renderings of Three Dimensional Pipe Test with scores of 0 (poor) through 3 (excellent).

evidence of three dimensionality. The clock should contain two of the following: circular face, the numbers 1 through 12, or symmetrical number placement. The daisy should be in the generally appropriate shape—a circular center with petals around it. The house should contain the basic elements of a house.

3—Excellent Given for perfect (or near perfect) representations of the items with all appropriate components, placement, and perspective. The house and flower pot should be clearly three dimensional.

Representative clinical examples of poor, fair, good, and excellent drawings are shown in Figures 7-8 to 7-10 to aid the examiner in rating each picture.

Block Designs

The following test, although important and often providing excellent clinical data, does require equipment other than paper and pencil, and is considered ancillary. The medical student may not have ready access to the materials necessary; the practicing clinical neurologist should and should utilize the test in the complete mental status examination.

Directions. The use of this test requires only four multicolored cubes (obtained from the suppliers of the WAIS or from many toy stores as Kohs blocks) and four stimulus designs which may be readily drawn with colored pens or pencils on pieces of heavy white paper. The stimulus designs should be accurately drawn in the approximate size of the design completed with blocks. The designs in Figure 7-11 are arranged in ascending order of difficulty; start with 1 for all patients and administer all designs in order. Take four blocks and say "These blocks are all alike. On some sides they are all red; on some, all white; and on some they are half red and half white. I would like you to take these blocks and make a design (or picture) that looks like this picture." If the patient fails to accurately reproduce Design 1, score his response as a failure and demonstrate the correct reproduction. Continue with each design in turn, being sure to mix up the blocks after each effort.

Scoring. Only perfect reproductions of the designs are considered correct. Rotations (either right-left or near-far) are scored as incorrect as are figure-ground (color) reversals. A score of 1 is given for each correctly reproduced design. Perfect reproductions of each design are expected in the normal individual.

Examples of commonly seen rotation, reversal, and "stringing out" errors are shown in Figure 7-12.

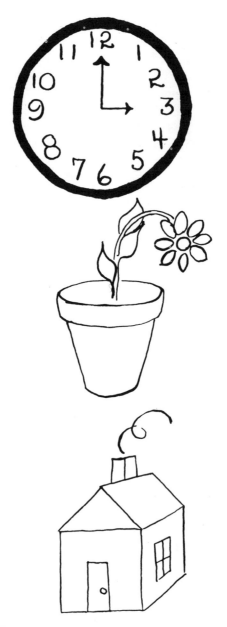

FIGURE 7-7. Test items for Drawings to Command Test. See text.

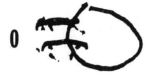

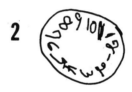

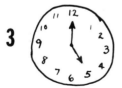

FIGURE 7-8. Renderings of Drawings to Command Test (clock) with scores of 0 (poor) through 3 (excellent).

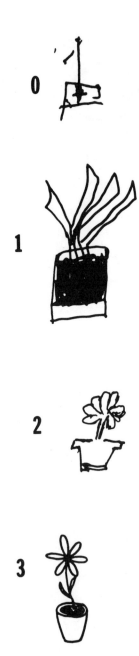

FIGURE 7-9. Renderings of Drawings to Command Test (flower pot) with scores of 0 (poor) through 3 (excellent).

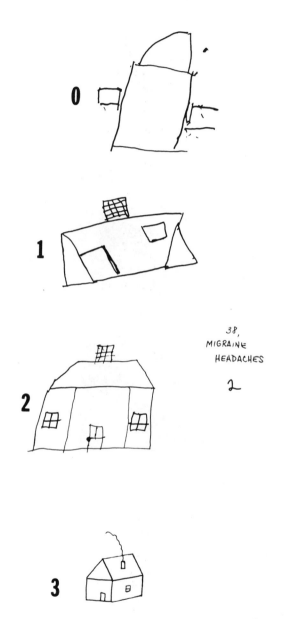

FIGURE 7-10. Renderings of Drawings to Command Test (house in perspective) with scores of 0 (poor) through 3 (excellent).

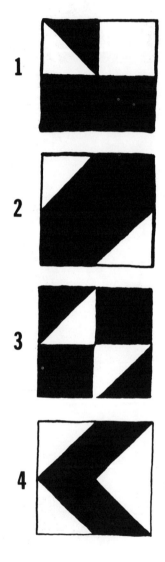

FIGURE 7-11. Test items for Block Designs Test. See text.

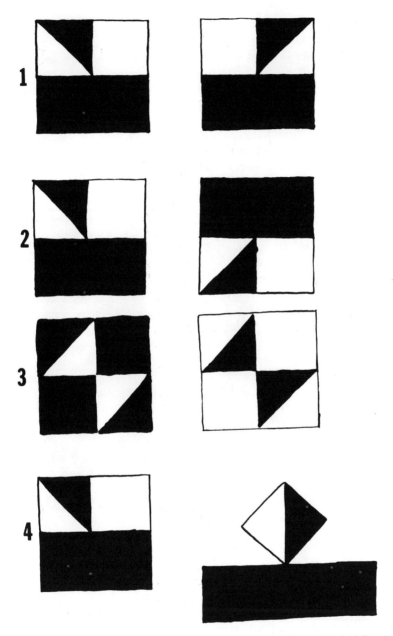

FIGURE 7-12. Examples of common errors on Block Designs Test. 1, Right-left rotation. 2, Near-far rotation. 3, Figure-ground reversal. 4, "Stringing out."

ANATOMY

The parietal lobes are the principle cortical areas involved in the visual motor integration of constructional tasks. Visual receptive areas of the occipital lobes and the motor areas of the frontal lobes are necessary for the completion of all the tests presented here but it is the association cortex of parietal lobes that is responsible for the complex integration. The actual localization of the various aspects of construction within the parietal lobes has not been possible but it is postulated[11] that visual stimuli is spread from primary sensory area 17 to contiguous secondary association areas 18 and 19 where perception is elaborated and compared to previous experience. The stimuli then spread to the tertiary association area of the inferior parietal lobule (areas 39 and 40) where associations are made between visual, auditory, and kinesthetic images. Most constructional tasks require primarily the kinesthetic analysis of the visual pattern. The kinesthetic images are then translated into motor patterns in the perirolandic cortex. Drawings to command require in addition an input from the auditory system. The premotor frontal association cortex would seem to be very important in these highly skilled fine motor tasks, but in fact, only a small percentage of patients with lesions restricted to the frontal lobes have constructional impairment. The parietal lobes seem to be the major areas involved in learning skilled movements, while the frontal motor areas appear more involved in the pure executive nature of the task. (A more extensive discussion of learned skilled movements is in the section on apraxia in Chap. 9).

CLINICAL IMPLICATIONS

If a nonretarded adult demonstrates constructional impairment on the tests outlined in this chapter, parietal lobe dysfunction can be strongly suspected. Though it has been shown that lesions in any quadrant of the brain can disrupt constructional performance, the incidence and severity of defects in patients with lesions restricted to the frontal lobes is small. Most constructional impairment is seen in patients with cortical damage posterior to the Rolandic fissure.

At one time it was felt that the right (nondominant) parietal lobe was actually dominant for constructional ability. Many studies have been carried out comparing the relative incidence and severity of constructional impairment in lesions of right and left hemispheres. These studies clearly demonstrate that performance can be defective with lesions in either parietal lobe. In general, right hemisphere lesions produce a higher incidence and greater severity of defect than do left hemisphere lesions.[3] What is certain is that constructional ability is not a function exclusive to the right parietal lobe.

Some subtle differences in the qualitative performance that are both interesting and possibly useful in clinical testing have been noted in right and left parietal lobe patients. On the block designs test, right lesioned patients frequently lose the basic outline of the design and "string out" the blocks.[9] This is shown in example 4, Figure 7-12. These patients tend to make scattered and fragmented drawings showing loss of spatial relations and orientation on the page. Left hemisphere lesioned patients show more coherent block designs with maintenance of external configuration but loss of accurate internal detail (example 3, Fig. 7-12). Their drawings tend to be simplifications of the model, lacking detail but with preserved general spatial relationships. Obvious differences in the performance of the two groups are not always seen and elaborate scoring schemes have often been designed to bring out the subtle differences. Such systems are interesting but probably not of practical significance to the bedside clinician. Thus constructional impairment strongly suggests parietal lobe pathology, but without very careful assessment of qualitative performance it is usually not possible using constructional tests alone to determine the side of the lesion in the individual patient. When a patient's constructional ability is grossly impaired, while verbal ability is relatively well maintained, right hemisphere dysfunction is strongly suggested.

Tumors and vascular accidents confined to the parietal lobes can show constructional impairment in the presence of a normal standard neurologic exam. This objective data of parietal dysfunction should lead the clinician to pursue his diagnostic evaluation.

The most dramatic examples of constructional impairment occur in patients with bilateral cortical disease. This is particularly well demonstrated in cerebral atrophy. Patients with Alzheimer's disease (by far the most common presenile dementia) and senile dementia regularly show constructional difficulty as one of the earliest signs of their disease.[14] The patient with the multiple infarct dementia seen in cerebral vascular disease will also show constructional impairment, but usually has other abnormal neurologic signs. Patients in confusional states from toxic or metabolic factors frequently have constructional impairment in the acute stage, but this is secondary to reversible physiologic disturbance of the cortex rather than structural damage. Since no permanent dysfunction is expected in these patients, the examiner must always be cautious interpreting any abnormalities found.

Because of the high incidence of constructional impairment in dementia, such tasks are very good organic screening tests in patients of advancing age who present with vague psychiatric or neurologic complaints.

Standard drawing and other constructional tests are not only useful in the detection of brain disease but also have been commonly used by psychologists to evaluate both the maturational stage of perceptual-motor development (constructional ability) and the presence of specific constructional problems in children. The ability to integrate visual stimuli and to construct or draw a reproduction is closely related to both chronologic and intellectual maturation in young children.[2, 6, 10] Errors in construction including poor integration of the parts, distortions or simplification, perseveration, and rotations are common early in development (5 to 7 years) and tend to decrease with age.[5] Relatively errorless performance on simple drawing tests is expected by age 10 to 12.[10] Measured intelligence tends to be relatively highly correlated with constructional performance in children,[10] while for adults of normal intelligence (e.g., above 85), IQ appears to have a limited effect upon constructional ability.[12] Both children and adults with significant mental deficiency tend to show inferior performance on most constructional tests.[4] Formal studies[15] have indicated that it is difficult using drawing tests to differentiate intellectually retarded (e.g., IQ below 70), but socially and vocationally independent adults from similar individuals with demonstrable brain damage.

As with any skilled motor coordination activity, both initial exposure and repeated practice have an effect upon the ability to reproduce paper and pencil designs or to complete block constructions. Social deprivation and a lack of academic experience do, therefore, have a detrimental effect upon constructional performance.

The physician using constructional tests as a part of the mental status examination must be cautious in interpreting the results of performance by patients with a history of retardation and/or a poor academic background. Placed in the proper interpretative context, however, we feel that drawings and other constructional tests may be fruitfully used with such patients.

A number of specific types of errors on constructional tests are generally accepted as almost pathognomonic of brain damage when made by a nonretarded patient above the age of ten years. The majority of these errors can be seen on both paper and pencil and block design tests. Of primary importance among these pathognomonic signs are the following:

1. The rotation by more than 45 degrees or the disorientation of the whole figure or a component of it on the background.

2. Perseveration or the repetition of the entire figure or a part of it.

3. Fragmentation of the design or the omission of parts of the figure.

4. Significant difficulty in integration or the placing of individual parts at the correct angles or location.

5. The substitution or addition of "dog ears" for angles on the drawn figure.

The occurrence of any of these errors should raise a strong question of brain dysfunction requiring more detailed evaluation.

SUMMARY

Constructional ability is a highly developed cortical integrative function that is primarily carried out in the parietal lobes. Drawings and block constructions are easily adminstered tests to evaluate this function. Impairment of constructional performance suggests disease of the posterior portions of the cerebral hemispheres, although occasionally anterior lesions also cause disturbance.

REFERENCES

1. Arrigoni, G., and De Renzi, E.: Constructional apraxia and hemispheric locus of lesions. Cortex 1:170, 1964.
2. Bender, E.: A visual motor gestalt test and its clinical use. American Orthopsychiatric Association, New York, 1938.
3. Benson, D. F., and Barton, M.: Disturbances in constructional ability. Cortex 6:19, 1970.
4. Benton, A.: Revised Visual Retention Test. The Psychological Corporation, New York, 1974.
5. Black, F. W.: Reversal and rotation errors by normal and retarded readers. Percept. Mot. Skills 36:895, 1973.
6. Frostig, M., Lefever, D., and Whittlesey, J.: A. developmental test of visual perception for evaluating normal and neurologically handicapped children. Percept. Mot. Skills 12:383, 1961.
7. Geschwind, N.: The apraxias: Neural mechanisms of disorders of learned movement. Am. Sci. 63:188, 1975.
8. Graham, F., and Kendall, B.: Memory for Designs Test. Psychological Test Specialists, Missoula, Mont., 1960.
9. Kaplan, E.: Personal communication. 1973.
10. Koppitz, E.: The Bender Gestalt Test for Young Children. 1964, Grune and Stratton, New York, 1964.
11. Luria, A.: The Working Brain. Basic Books, New York, 1973.
12. Pascal, G., and Suttell, B.: The Bender Gestalt Test. Grune and Stratton, New York, 1951.
13. Piercy, M., Hecaen, H., and Ajuriaguerra, J.: Constructional apraxia associated with unilateral lesions: Left and right cases compared. Brain 83:232, 1960.
14. Sjörgen, T., Sjörgen, T., and Lindgren, A. G. H.: Morbus Alzheimer and Morbus Pick: A Genetic, Clinical, and Pathoanatomical Study. Munksgaard, Copenhagen, 1952.

15. Strub, R. L., and Black, F. W.: Constructional apraxia: A frequent finding in the low IQ normal population. Paper presented at the American Academy of Neurology, May 1, 1975, Miami.
16. Warrington, E.: Constructional apraxia, in Vinken, P., and Bruyn, G. (eds.): Handbook of Clinical Neurology, Volume 4, Disorders of Speech, Perception and Symbolic Behavior. American Elsevier, Amsterdam, 1969, pp. 67–83.

CHAPTER 8

Higher Cognitive Functions

Attention, language, and memory are the basic processes which serve as building blocks for the development of higher intellectual abilities. These basic functions are necessary, but not sufficient in and of themselves, to execute more complex cognitive functions. By use of the term higher cognitive functions we refer to the highest level of human intellectual functioning that can be readily assessed by formal testing methods. Included within this category of functions are the manipulation of well learned material, abstract thinking, arithmetic computations, and so forth. These are complex neuropsychologic functions which are predicated upon the integrity and interaction of more basic processes.

Because they do represent the most advanced stages of intellectual development, the higher cognitive functions are often highly susceptible to neurologic disease. The evaluation of these functions in the mental status examination may often demonstrate the early effects of cortical damage before the more basic processes of attention, language, and memory are impaired. The individual's ability to perform effectively within his environment is determined in a large part by an adequacy in carrying out these higher order functions. Accordingly, an assessment of the patient's performance in these areas will provide useful information concerning his social and vocational prognosis.

EVALUATION

There are many ways to evaluate the higher cognitive functions: most intelligence tests are largely based upon assessments of these functions. In general, the higher cognitive functions may be categorized in the following hierarchical groupings: (1) the fund of acquired information or store of knowledge, (2) the manipulation of old knowledge (e.g., calculations or problem solving), (3) social awareness and judgment, and (4) abstract thinking (e.g., the interpretation of unfamiliar proverbs or the completion of conceptual series). The store of basic acquired information is most efficiently assessed by simple verbal tests of vocabulary, general information, and comprehension. Specific examples of these kinds of tests may be seen on any basic intelligence test (e.g., WAIS Vocabulary, Information, Picture Completion). General intelligence, education, and social exposure are closely related to performance on these tasks and the results of any evaluation must be interpreted in the light of this background information. The manipulation of old knowledge is a more active process which involves both an intact fund of general information and the ability to apply this information to new or unfamiliar situations. Questions concerning social comprehension and calculation ability may be used to assess this function. Social awareness may be evaluated by questions concerning the knowledge of environmental situations (e.g., What should a person do if he sees smoke or fire in a grocery store?). Social judgment is a more complex function including both the basic knowledge of social situations, the socially appropriate response in such situations, and the ability to personally apply the correct response when faced with a real situation. Because of the real nature of social judgment, it is difficult to assess validly in an abstract test situation. The patient who matter of factly states that he would calmly inform the manager of smoke or fire in the store when asked the question in the confines of an office or hospital bed may act very differently when faced with the actual situation! Therefore, data concerning the patient's social judgment is best obtained by history from family or other informants who have witnessed his actual performance in dealing with day to day events. An alternative possibility, albeit a somewhat cumbersome and inefficient procedure, is to place the patient in actual, but experimental situations requiring an immediate appropriate social response. This method of evaluation is likely to be impractical except in research settings, thus the social history is recommended for practical purposes. Abstract thinking, which is perhaps the highest level of cognition, may be readily assessed in the formal test situation by the use of proverbs, conceptual series, or analogy interpretation.

The following tests are recommended to evaluate a spectrum of the relevant higher cognitive functions.

Fund of Information

Directions. The following questions provide a reasonable estimate of the patient's store of knowledge or fund of general information. They are presented in order of increasing difficulty and should be administered in this order for all patients. If it is obvious from history or interview that the patient is of above average intelligence, some of the less difficult questions may be omitted. Continue to ask questions until completion of the test or until the patient has failed three successive questions. If the patient's response is unclear, ask him to explain more fully. The examiner may repeat the question if necessary, but should not paraphrase the question or spell or explain words unfamiliar to the patient.

Test Items	*Acceptable Responses*
1. How many weeks are in the year?	52
2. Why do people have lungs?	Transfer oxygen from air to blood. Provide oxygen to body.
3. Name four men who have been president of the US since 1940.	Any appropriate presidents.
ʄ 4. Where is Luxembourg?	Europe
✗5. How far is it from New York to Los Angeles?	Any answer between 2,300 and 2,700 miles.
6. Why are light colored clothes cooler in the summer than dark colored clothes?	Light colored clothes reflect heat from the sun, while dark colored clothes absorb heat.
7. What is the capitol of Spain?	Madrid
8. What causes rust?	Oxidation. A chemical reaction of metal, oxygen, and moisture.
✗ 9. Who wrote the Odyssey?	Homer
✗10. What is the Acropolis?	Site of the Parthenon in Athens.

Scoring. The acceptable response for each question is provided above. The patient's answer must be exact or very closely approximate to the acceptable response. In our experience, the average patient with an adequate educational background should answer a minimum of six questions appropriately. Less adequate performance is indicative of an impaired fund of general information and is suspicious of retardation, limited social and educational exposure, or significant dementia. Conversely, more adequate performance suggests above average intelligence and education.

Proverb Interpretation

Directions. The ability to interpret proverbs accurately requires an intact fund of general information, the ability to apply this knowledge to unfamiliar situations, and the ability to think in the abstract. The following proverbs are presented in ascending order of difficulty. Tell the patient, "I am going to read you a saying which you may or may not have heard before. Explain in your own words what the saying means." Read each proverb exactly as written. Do not paraphrase or otherwise explain the proverb. Continue only until the patient fails on two successive proverbs.

Test Items.
1. Rome wasn't built in a day.
2. A drowning man will clutch at a straw.
3. A golden hammer breaks an iron door.
4. The hot coal burns, the cold one blackens.

Scoring. The primary scoring criterion for proverb interpretation is the degree of abstraction demonstrated by the patient in explaining the proverb. It is helpful to rate the quality of the patient's response to each proverb. To aid the examiner, examples of abstract (2 points), semiabstract (1 point), and concrete (0 points) responses to each proverb are provided below:

1. Rome wasn't built in a day.

0—concrete	"It took a long time to build Rome."
	"You can't build cities overnight."
	"Some things you can't do in one day."
1—semiabstract	"Don't do things too fast."
	"You have to be patient and careful."
	"Can't learn everything right away."
2—abstract	"Great things take time to achieve."
	"If something is worth doing, it is worth doing it carefully."
	"It takes time to do things well."

2. A drowning man will clutch at a straw.

0—concrete	"Don't let go when you're in the water."
	"He's trying to save himself."
	"That guy will grab anything."
1—semiabstract	"Self-preservation is important."
	"It's a last resort."
	"Nobody wants to die."
2—abstract	"A man in trouble will try anything to get out of it."
	"A person who is losing will use almost any method to get ahead."
	"If sufficiently desperate, a man will try anything."

3. A golden hammer breaks an iron door.

0—concrete	"Gold can't break iron!"

	"Gold is too soft to break a door."
	"Hammers can break down doors."
1—semiabstract	"Money wins everything."
	"The harder something is, the more you have to work to get it."
2—abstract	"Vitrue conquers all."
	"If you have sufficient knowledge, you can accomplish even the most difficult."

4. The hot coal burns, the cold one blackens.

0—concrete	"Hot coals will burn you and leave it black."
	"Hot coals get black when they're cold."
1—semiabstract	"You can get trouble from both."
	"Getting burned and dirty are both bad."
2—abstract	"Extremes of anything can be bad."
	"There may be bad aspects to things that appear good."
	"One should be careful and not impetuous in any situation."

Concrete responses are pathologic in all but the retarded and/or illiterate patient. The average patient should provide abstract interpretations to at least two proverbs and minimally semiabstract responses to the remaining proverbs. Often uneducated patients will initially give a concrete response, but can give abstract interpretations when specifically asked if there is another way of explaining the proverb. Such cued responses should be scored 1 as a semiabstract response. A total score of less than five on proverb interpretation is suspicious. Any concrete response or an absence of some abstract responses should suggest an impairment of abstract ability.

Similarities

Directions. Verbal similarities require the patient to explain the basic similarity between two overtly different objects or situations. Similarities is a test of verbal abstract ability which requires the analysis of relationships, the formation of verbal concepts, and logical thinking in the abstract sphere. The following tests items are presented in ascending order of difficulty. Tell the patient, "I am going to tell you some pairs of objects. Please tell me how they are similar or alike. Each pair is alike in some way." Present the first item pair. If the patient provides the appropriate abstract response, say, "Good," and proceed with the next item. If the patient mentions a difference between the items, fails to respond, or states that they are different, score the item 0, provide the appropriate response, and continue with item 2. Give no help on succeeding items.

Test Items.
1. Turnip—Cauliflower
2. Desk—Bookcase
3. Poem—Novel
4. Horse—Apple

Scoring. The response for each item pair may be scored for adequacy. Two points should be given for any abstract similarity or general classification which is highly pertinent for both items in the pair. One point should be given for responses indicating specific properties pertinent to both items in the pair and which constitute a relevant similarity. A score of 0 is given when the response reflects specific properties of one member of the pair, differences, generalizations which are not pertinent to the item pair, and failures to respond. Examples of 2, 1, and 0 point responses are provided below:

1. Turnip—Cauliflower

    2 points: Vegetables

    1 point: Food; they grow in the ground; to eat.

    0 points: Buy in the store; have calories; wash them.

2. Desk—Bookcase

    2 points: Articles of furniture.

    1 point: Household objects; in the living room; put book on them.

    0 points: Made out of wood; sit at a desk and put books in the bookcase.

3. Poem—Novel

    2 points: Artistic works; works of art; creative expression; literary works.

    1 point: Write them both; symbolic; tell stories; express feelings.

    0 points: Famous things; study them in school; people like them.

4. Horse—Apple

    2 points: Living things; God's living objects.

    1 point: Both grow; both are food; both need food; part of nature.

    0 points: Horses eat apples; one is big and one is small; we use them.

The nonretarded patient with a normal educational background should obtain a score of at least 4 on this test. Any one concrete (0 point) response or score of less than 4 is strongly suggestive of reduced general intelligence or impaired abstract ability. Concrete responses are virtually pathognomonic of dysfunction. In general, performance on this test should be compatible with performance on the Fund of Information test and on the Proverb Interpretation test. If Similarities and Fund of Information performance are equally impaired, this is suggestive of retardation or educational deprivation rather than a specific deficit in abstract thinking.

Calculations

Directions. Calculations are complex neuropsychologic functions which involve the somewhat distinct components of (a) rote tables (e.g., addition, subtraction, and multiplication), (b) the basic arithmetic concepts of carrying and borrowing, (c) recognition of the signs $(+, -, \times,$ and $\div)$, and (d) correct spatial alignment for written calculations. Because these components of calculations may be disturbed in isolation in some neurologic conditions, they are assessed separately in this section. When evaluating calculations, it is important to require the patient to actually calculate and not to merely recite rote tables (e.g., $4 + 4 = 8$, or $3 \times 5 = 15$). This allows the observation of many different types of errors and provides additional clinical data which are important for a description of the nature of the deficit and also for providing neuroanatomic implications. Performance on calculation is, of course, closely related to educational experience. Tell the patient, "We are now going to do some arithmetic examples. Some will be familiar to you and some will not. Try your best on each one."

Verbal Rote Examples

Read each example in a clear voice in the following form: "What is 4 and 6?" Record the patient's response.

1. Addition:

$4 + 6 = (10)$
$7 + 9 = (16)$
$2 + 5 = (7)$
$5 + 8 = (13)$

2. Subtraction:

$8 - 5 = (3)$
$11 - 4 = (7)$
$17 - 9 = (8)$
$7 - 5 = (2)$

3. Multiplication:

$4 \times 8 = (32)$
$7 \times 7 = (49)$
$8 \times 3 = (24)$
$9 \times 7 = (63)$

4. Division:

$9 \div 3 = (3)$
$12 \div 6 = (2)$
$56 \div 8 = (7)$
$124 \div 4 = (31)$

Verbal Complex Examples

Read each example in the following form only once: "What is 8 and 13?" Allow only 10 seconds for a response; a failure to respond within that time, even if a correct response it ultimately given, is scored as a failure. Record the patient's response.

1. Addition:

$$8 + 13 = (21)$$
$$14 + 17 = (31)$$
$$23 + 39 = (62)$$

2. Subtraction:

$$31 - 19 = (12)$$
$$17 - 12 = (5)$$
$$43 - 38 = (5)$$

3. Multiplication:

$$17 \times 3 = (51)$$
$$21 \times 5 = (105)$$
$$14 \times 9 = (126)$$

4. Division:

$$84 \div 6 = (14)$$
$$72 \div 3 = (24)$$
$$128 \div 8 = (16)$$

Written Complex Examples

Provide the patient with the following written examples and ask him to complete the example. To preclude problems of distractability and perseveration, it is useful to provide each example on individual cards or to write each new example after the patient completes the previous example. Examples written on a single sheet of paper should be widely separated. Allow only 20 seconds for completion of each example. A failure to complete the example within 20 seconds is scored as a failure. Record the patient's response, including problems in alignment.

1. Addition:

$$17 + 29 = \quad (46)$$
$$108 + 79 = \quad (187)$$
$$1,004 + 19 = (1,023)$$

2. Subtraction:

$$648 - 51 = (597)$$
$$605 - 86 = (519)$$
$$1,208 - 949 = (259)$$

3. Multiplication:

$$68 \times 7 = \quad (476)$$
$$108 \times 36 = \quad (3,888)$$
$$1,482 \times 64 = (94,848)$$

4. Division:

$$348 \div 6 = \quad (58)$$
$$559 \div 43 = \quad (13)$$
$$3,654 \div 29 = (126)$$

Scoring. Each response should be scored as correct or incorrect. By comparing performance on each computation subtest, it is possible to determine the patient's overall level of calculation ability and his area of adequacy and deficit (e.g., intact rote tables, but unable to complete complex verbally presented examples). Errors specific to a particular aspect of computation (e.g., division) and to a modality of presentation (e.g., intact performance on verbally presented items and impaired performance on written examples) should be noted. Errors involving borrowing (e.g., 8 + 13 or 14 × 9) and alignment on written examples should be recorded.

No norms are currently available for this clinical test of calculation ability. If a more objective measure of arithmetic is needed, the examiner should refer to a standard achievement test such as the Wide Range Achievement Test.[5]

Conceptual Series Completion

Directions. The Conceptual Series Completion is another test of verbal abstraction, the ability to solve unfamiliar and complex verbal problems, and to reason at a high level. Tell the patient, "I am going to show you some numbers, letters, or words in series. Each series will be incomplete and needs an additional word, letter, or number to complete it. Each dash (—) calls for either a number or letter to be filled in. Take each item in order, but if you don't understand it, don't spend too much time on any one item." The following sequences are presented to the patient in written form, either on a standard form prepared beforehand by the examiner or written on a sheet of paper by the examiner.

Test Items	*Correct Response*
1. 1 4 7 10 __ __	13
2. AZ BY CX D __	W
3. tote to snow on spun up stab __ __	at
4. elephant 87654321 plant 5732 lap __ __ __	735

Scoring. Each response is scored as correct or incorrect using the above scoring criteria. No unique or original interpretations of the correct response are allowed. The average patient should be capable of completing at least two of the four examples correctly. Less adequate performance is indicative of impaired ability to think in the abstract or to reason verbally.

Anatomy

The higher cognitive functions are primarily cortically localized. They are not, however, functions which have been well localized in the way that language or constructional ability have. Abstract thinking, the ability to manipulate old knowledge, calculation ability, and similar functions are probably widely represented in the cortex. Because of this diffuse representation, an impairment of these functions results from lesions located in various parts of the cortex. Impairment is particularly prominent in widespread bilateral disease (e.g., dementia).

It is likely that these higher cognitive functions are more posteriorly than frontally localized. Although a "loss of abstraction" has been traditionally considered an early sign of frontal lobe dysfunction and was described in patients following frontal lobectomies,[6] underlying defects of attention, memory, and perseveration typically account for the deficits in higher cognition.[4] In a comprehensive review of the literature concerned with the interaction of frontal lesions and cognitive functioning (higher cognitive functions), Teuber[7] concluded that such lesions generally affect intelligence less than lesions located in the more posterior areas of the brain. Black[1] also documented the differential effects of frontal and nonfrontal unilateral lesions upon cognitive functions. This study again verified that the higher cognitive functions are primarily impaired with posterior lesions.

Verbal reasoning and abstraction are primarily dominant hemisphere functions with very close connections with the dominant language structures. Thus, dominant hemisphere lesions frequently interfere with these high level verbal manipulations.

Impaired performance on calculations may be seen with brain lesions which are bilateral or unilateral on either the right or left side.[2] Lesions in somewhat different areas of the brain may cause different types of impaired calculation ability (dyscalculia). Left hemisphere lesions in the right handed patient typically result in more severe impairment of calculations than do corresponding lesions of the nondominant hemisphere. A significant dyscalculia often accompanies an aphasic disturbance secondary to a left hemisphere lesion. Similarly, dyscalculia is a significant component of the Gerstmann syndrome (described in Chap. 9) which is secondary to a dominant parietal lobe lesion. Specific calculation defects ascribed to focal frontal, temporal, parietal, and occipital lesions have been described.[3] The utility of such overschematization for the typical examiner is questionable, however. Impaired calculation ability due to focal lesions in the parietal lobes appears to be more common or at least the subject of more frequent research investigation. This type of disorder is characterized by a loss of the ability to understand the meaning of numbers and numerical concepts (e.g., larger or smaller) and the inability to align numbers correctly on the page due to visual spatial deficits. The malalignment in complex computations can often be the most striking feature in the dyscalculia seen with parietal lobe lesions.

CLINICAL IMPLICATIONS

Deficits in higher cognitive functions are most frequently seen in patients with widespread brain disease of any etiology. These deficits may often be the first sign of deterioration in progressive brain disease such as Alzheimer's disease or subacute sclerosing panencephalitis.

Focal dominant parietal lobe lesions may demonstrate defects in the verbally mediated functions and must be considered in the differential diagnosis in any patient presenting with a loss of abstract ability or impaired calculations. As discussed previously, lesions of the frontal lobe typically do not interfere with the fund of knowledge, abstract thinking, and problem solving unless other more basic deficits are also present (e.g., perseveration or aphasia). Conversely, social awareness and judgment in social situations is often impaired with large frontal lesions.

Significant functional disease, particularly schizophrenia, may result in impaired abstracting ability. Although the concreteness of the schizophrenic is frequently different in nature from that of the organic patient (e.g., a symbolic interpretation incorporating the patient's delusions), at times the deficit may be indistinguishable from an organic concreteness. Any significant psychiatric disorder of either a psychotic or neurotic nature will hamper the patient's ability to attend to the examiner and to perform on any test of higher cognitive function.

Because of the close relationship between higher cognitive functions and general intelligence, mental retardation from whatever cause will result in impaired performance on these tests. Educational deprivation will similarly result in substandard performance which is not of diagnostic significance. Accordingly, performance on the tests of higher cognitive function must be interpreted within the context of both educational background and premorbid intelligence. The test of fund of information provides a reasonable estimate of current intellectual functioning which may be combined with data from history to furnish this background information.

SUMMARY

Higher cognitive functions are measures of the patient's reasoning and problem solving abilities. These functions are often impaired early in brain disease and thereby offer an effective measure for detecting brain disease in patients with relatively intact performance in other areas such as language, constructional ability, and memory. Any deficits will be reflected in the patient's inability to function effectively within his environment. Thus, an evaluation of these functions will aid in making a valid social and vocational prognosis.

REFERENCES

1. Black, W.: Cognitive deficits in patients with unilateral war-related frontal lobe lesions. J. Clin. Psychol. 32:366, 1976.
2. Critchley, M.: The Parietal Lobes. Edward Arnold & Co., London, 1953.
3. Grewel, F.: Alcalculias, in Vinken, P., and Bruyn, G. (eds): Handbook of Clinical

Neurology, Vol. 4, Disorders of Speech, Perception, and Symbolic Behavior. American Elsevier, New York, 1969, pp. 181-194.

4. Hecaen, H., and Albert, M.: Disorders of mental functioning related to frontal lobe pathology, in Benson, F ., and Blumer, D. (eds.): Psychiatric Aspects of Neurologic Disease. Grune & Stratton, New York, 1975, pp. 137-149.

5. Jastak, J., and Jastak, S.: The Wide Range Achievement Test. Guidance Associates, Wilmington, 1965.

6. Rylander, G.: Mental Changes After Excision of Cerebral Tissue. Einar Munsgaar, Copenhagen, 1943.

7. Teuber, H.-L.: The riddle of frontal lobe function in man, in Warrren, J., and Akert, K. (eds.): The Frontal Granular Cortex and Behavior. McGraw-Hill, New York, 1964, pp. 410-444.

CHAPTER 9

Related Cortical Functions

There is a group of specific cortical functions that has been of great interest to neurologists and psychologists. Most of these functions are related to high level motor and sensory processing. Apraxia is an example of a high level motor disturbance, while visual agnosia is a high level perceptual disturbance. These functions are of some utility in cerebral localization and are of considerable research interest to neurobehaviorists. Because each of these related cortical functions is relatively discrete, a complete discussion of terminology, evaluation, and clinical implications of each will be presented separately.

APRAXIA

Apraxia is an acquired disorder of learned movements that cannot be accounted for by elementary disturbances of strength coordination, sensation, or lack of comprehension or attention.[19] Many textbooks refer to apraxia as a defect in motor planning. Both definitions indicate that apraxia is not a low level motor disturbance, but a defect in the integrative steps that precede skilled or learned movements. Different types of apraxia have been described based upon the complexity and nature of the task performed. There is a motor disturbance that is seen in the limb opposite a cortical lesion that is characterized by clumsiness or involuntary grasp reflexes.[11] This disturbance has been called a limb-kinetic apraxia. As these patients have difficulty with basic motor control and display abnormal reflexes, their movements do not meet the classical definition of apraxia.

Ideomotor Apraxia

Ideomotor apraxia is the most common type of apraxia. Patients with this form of apraxia fail to accurately carry out previously learned motor acts to the examiner's command. Impairment can be seen in buccofacial, upper or lower limb, or trunkal musculature. Failure to carry out such commands as, "Show me how you blow out a match," or "Drink through a straw" are called buccofacial apraxia. Difficulty with arm or leg commands such as flipping a coin, saluting, or kicking a ball are called limb apraxia, and difficulty with trunkal commands such as "Bow," "Swing a baseball bat," or "Stand like a boxer," is called an apraxia of whole body movements.

Evaluation. There is a hierarchy of difficulty in carrying out these ideomotor tasks. The most difficult level requires that the patient carry out the action to verbal command (e.g., "Show me how to flip a coin."). This movement must be mimicked without the coin and without any nonverbal cues from the examiner. If the patient fails at this level, the examiner performs the action and asks the patient to imitate him. Imitation is easier for most patients with apraxia. If he again fails, the patient is provided with the real object and again asked to follow the command. Use of the actual object is the easiest task for the apraxic and many, but not all, of the patients failing on verbal command and imitation will succeed with the concrete task using the real object. The presence of the object gives the patient additional visual and proprioceptive cues that facilitate performance. There are innumerable possible commands when evaluating praxis. The following are examples that will frequently elicit apraxic movements.

Buccofacial Commands

Commands	*Errors*
"Show me how to:"	
1. "Blow out a match"	Difficulty giving a short controlled exhalation, saying "blow," inhaling, difficulty maintaining appropriate mouth posture
2. "Protrude the tongue"	Unable to stick out tongue, tongue moves in mouth but tends to push against front teeth and not protude
3. "Drink through a straw"	Unable to sustain a pucker, blowing instead of drawing through the straw, random mouthing movements

In testing buccofacial praxis, the patient can often cue himself considerably by pretending to have the object (match or straw) in his hand. This self-cuing facilitates performance and should be discouraged by gently restraining the patient's hands.

Limb Commands

Commands	Errors
"Show me how to:"	
1. "Salute"	Hand over head, hand waving, improper position of hand
2. "Use a toothbrush"	Failure to show proper grip, failure to open mouth, grossly missing the mouth, using finger to pick teeth, not allowing adequate distance for shaft of toothbrush
3. "Flip a coin"	Movements mimicking tossing the coin into the air with an open hand, suppinating or pronating the hand as though turning a doorknob, flexing of the arm without flipping thumb against finger
4. "Hammer a nail"	Move hand back and forth horizontally, pound with fist, uncertainty of grip
5. "Comb your hair"	Using fingers as teeth of comb, smoothing the hair, inexact hand movements
6. "Snap your fingers"	Extension of fingers with patting movements, tapping finger on thumb, sliding finger off thumb with insufficient force
7. "Kick a ball"	Stamping foot, pushing foot along floor, lateral foot movements
8. "Crush out a cigarette"	Stamping foot, kicking, tapping foot on floor

There are occasions in which apraxia will be found unilaterally. Accordingly, commands should be alternated between left and right limbs. Do not have the patient do the same command sequentially with both hands as visual self-cuing will improve performance on the second trial.

Whole Body Commands

Commands	Errors
"Show me how to:"	
1. "Stand like a boxer"	Awkward arm position, hands at side
2. "Swing a baseball bat"	Difficulty in placing both hands together, chopping movements
3. "Bow"	Any inappropriate trunkal movement

Clinical Implications. The ability to perform skilled movements on verbal command is closely associated with the language functions of the dominant hemisphere. Since adequate verbal comprehension is a prerequisite to praxis testing, the area A (Fig. 9-1) must be intact. Once the command is understood, the information spreads to the contiguous supramarginal gyrus (area B, Fig. 9-1) where the words (e.g., "flip a coin") are associated with the kinesthetic memories present in the post-Rolandic parietal cortex. These sensory memories of the movement are then transferred along pathway C to the premotor area D where memory for motor patterns is evoked. The premotor area then directs the pyramidal neurons in the motor strip (area E), to actually perform the action. A lesion at any point along this pathway can cause an ideomotor apraxia. Most patients with lesions in this section of the dominant hemisphere will also be aphasic. Accordingly, praxis testing must be very carefully done to insure that a comprehension deficit is not responsible for the impaired performance.

The above paragraph outlines the pathways for praxis in the right hand (controlled by the left motor area). It has been recognized that the apraxic patient also has an apraxia with his left hand. Figure 9-2 illustrates that a command to the right motor cortex for innervation of the left hand is transferred from the left premotor area D_1 to the right premotor area D_2 via the anterior callosal fibers F_1. Any interruption of this pathway will render the left hand apraxic.[18,19] This is often called a sympathetic dyspraxia[17] and can be readily demonstrated in the intact

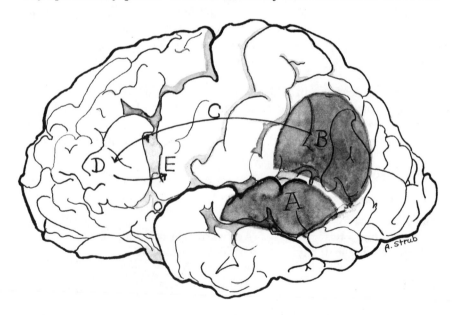

FIGURE 9-1

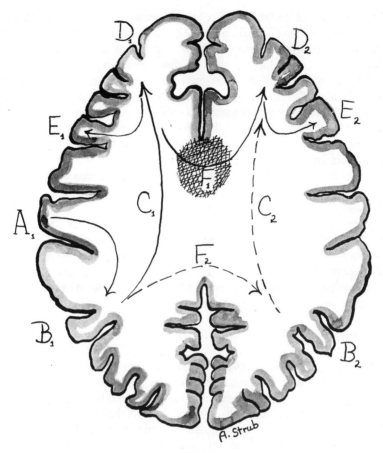

FIGURE 9-2

left hand of Broca's aphasics with right hemiplegia. Lesions of the anterior corpus callosum F_1 (Fig. 9-2) will cause an isolated apraxia of the left hand; motor and praxis functions of the right hand are intact.[21] The posterior callosal pathway F_2-C_2 which could theoretically transmit the praxis information to the right premotor area (area D_2) obviously does not. Lesions of the right hemisphere almost never result in an apraxia of either hand.[10]

This anatomic model has been verified clinically and pathologically and firmly establishes that the hemisphere dominant for language is also dominant for learning skilled movements.[19] This dominant hemisphere superiority is obvious because most individuals have a strong hand preference for writing, throwing, and so forth. Since a lesion of the dominant hemisphere causes an apraxia in both hands, it is apparent that the dominant hemisphere exerts a continual guiding role on movements originating from the nondominant hemisphere.

123

Not all apraxics demonstrate a similar degree and type of impaired performance. Some will fail completely on command, yet perform perfectly on imitation (even when comprehension of the command is adequate). Such patients have a type of disconnection syndrome in which verbal input is literally disconnected from motor areas. Visual input is relayed quickly to the motor areas and the patient can imitate without difficulty. Most apraxic patients who fail on command, however, also have difficulty with imitation. There are some patients with ideomotor apraxia whose disorder is sufficiently severe that they will fail on verbal command, imitation, and in the use of real objects.

Whole body commands are frequently carried out correctly in the presence of obvious limb apraxia. They can often be accurately carried out by patients with severe auditory comprehension deficits. The reason for the relative sparing of performance involving whole body commands is unclear, but may be due to the fact that these axial movements are under the control of the extrapyramidal system. The extrapyramidal system is much more widespread cortically than the pyramidal system and cannot be as easily disrupted as the more discrete pyramidal system which controls distal limb movements.[19]

Ideational Apraxia

Ideational apraxia is a higher order disturbance of complex motor planning than is seen in ideomotor apraxia. It refers to a breakdown in performance on a task involving a series of separate steps as folding a letter, placing it in an envelope, sealing it, and then placing a stamp on it. The patient is able to perform each individual step of the task in isolation (e.g., folding the paper), but is unable to integrate the parts accurately to complete the sequence. The patients seem to have lost the overall concept of how to go about completing the task. Some investigators define an ideational apraxia as any difficulty in manipulating real objects.[13] We feel that difficulty with object use in simple limb commands (e.g., inability to flip an actual coin) represents a severe ideomotor limb apraxia and not an ideational apraxia.

Evaluation. Several simple tasks are used to demonstrate an ideational apraxia.

Tasks	Errors
1. Folding a letter, placing it in an envelope, sealing it, and placing a stamp on the envelope	Turning paper around without being able to fold it, folding improperly, licking the wrong side of stamp or envelope, inability to place paper in envelope
2. Placing candle in holder, taking match out of box,	Placing candle in holder wick down, inability to place candle in holder, ina-

lighting candle, and blowing out match	bility to get match out of box, inability to open or close matchbox, striking match on candle, striking wrong end of match, striking candle, blowing out candle and not match
3. Opening toothpaste, taking brush from holder, and placing paste on brush	Removing cap from toothpaste and placing cap on brush, putting paste in brush holder, placing brush back in holder with paste on it

In each of these tasks the patient can usually carry out each part of the series perfectly (e.g., striking a match or brushing teeth), but he cannot coordinate the individual movements to complete the sequence.

Clinical Implications. Ideational apraxia is a complex disability that is usually seen in patients with bilateral brain disease. Any diffuse cortical disease, especially those effecting the parietal lobes, may result in an ideational apraxia. Although the patient fails on a specific task (e.g., lighting a candle), it is obvious from watching his performance that his failure is the result of a number of cognitive deficits. Many patients have elements of ideomotor apraxia and almost all have some degree of constructional impairment and spatial disorientation. Memory is frequently faulty and auditory comprehension diminished. One interesting element in the performance of patients with ideational apraxia is their apparent inability to recognize the use of objects. This failure to recognize object use has been called an object agnosia and may be illustrated by the patient who attempts to light a candle by striking it on the matchbox. The ability to do serial ordering is also impaired and the complex multistep task becomes a confusing group of discrete parts with no logical sequential relationship. The ambiguity and incongruity of the formal test situation also is confusing. The patient does not quite understand exactly what he is supposed to do when the doctor brings out a toothbrush and toothpaste and pushes it benignly toward the patient!

Neuropsychologically, ideational apraxia is the culmination of many significant cognitive deficits. Clinically, it results in the patient's inability to manipulate his environment. He cannot cook a meal, make a bed, light a cigarette, put a record on the phonograph, or do any of the dozens of everyday activities that we all take for granted. Ideational apraxia is not a finding seen in isolation, but is associated with widespread intellectual deterioration.

RIGHT-LEFT DISORIENTATION

Right-left orientation is traditionally defined as the ability to distinguish right from left on self and in the environment (e.g., on the examiner's body).

This ability is both a capacity for spatial orientation[7] and the application of the verbal labels "right" and "left" to the respective sides.[22] Right-left disorientation may be developmental in nature or may result from either focal or diffuse brain lesions. Although this disorder is interesting and may combine with other deficits to produce the Gerstmann syndrome (to be discussed later in this chapter), it is of limited clinical utility when seen in isolation.

Evaluation. The following outline which is in ascending order of difficulty may be used to test for right-left disorientation.

1. Identification on self
   a. Show me your right foot.
   b. Show me your left hand.
2. Crossed commands on self
   a. With your right hand touch your left shoulder.
   b. With your left hand touch your right ear.
3. Identification on examiner (with examiner facing patient)
   a. Point to my left knee.
   b. Point to my right elbow.
4. Crossed commands on examiner (with examiner facing patient)
   a. With your right hand point to my left eye.
   b. With your left hand point to my left foot.

There is no well established scoring system for the evaluation and interpretation of specific performance on these tasks; most normal persons will successfully accomplish all items without difficulty.

Clinical Implications. If right-left disorientation is present, it is important to determine if the patient was ever capable of adequately performing such tasks. As previously mentioned, right-left disorientation may be developmental in nature and may also be associated with reduced general intellectual ability.

Aphasic patients may fail on right-left commands because of their primary language disorder. Anomia can cause confusion in the use of the labels "right" and "left." Deficits in auditory retention will interfere with performance on complex commands.

Thus far, clinical and neuropathologic case studies have failed to demonstrate an association between right-left disorientation and any circumscribed brain lesion.[15] If an acquired disorder of right-left orientation is present, the lesion will generally be located in the parietotemporo-occipital region of the dominant hemisphere.[23] In our clinical experience, right-left disorientation is infrequent with lesions restricted to the nondominant hemisphere. This is also substantiated by Critchley's review.[7]

FINGER AGNOSIA

Finger agnosia is the inability to recognize, name, and point to individual fingers on one's self and on others.[16] This disorder may be most readily demonstrated in reference to the index, middle, and ring fingers.[7] Finger agnosia is similar to right-left orientation in that it may be developmental in nature or may result from either diffuse or focal brain disease. Its clinical utility for localization of cerebral lesions is relatively limited.

Evaluation

Evaluation of this function can by very extensive, however, this is probably not justified for practical purposes. A brief screening should suffice. Patients must have adequate auditory comprehension and know or be capable of learning the names of the fingers (thumb, index or pointing finger, middle finger, ring finger and little finger).

1. Identify Named Fingers on Examiner's Hand
Directions. The examiner's hand should be placed in various positions (i.e., palm down on the table facing patient, hand held vertical in air with palm facing patient, and hand horizontal in air with palm facing examiner). The examiner should say, "Point to my middle finger," etc.

2. Verbally Identify (Name) Fingers on Self and Examiner
Directions. The patient's and examiner's hands should be placed in the various positions as described above. The examiner points to the patient's index finger and says, "What is the name of this finger?" etc.

Clinical Implications
Patients with finger agnosia usually have lesions of the dominant hemisphere.[25] Left handed patients or those with strong family histories of left handedness may exhibit finger agnosia with lesions of either hemisphere. Parieto-occipital lesions tend to predominant among those causing finger agnosia.[29]

With more diffuse disease, finger agnosia may be seen as a concomitant of aphasia, apraxia, right-left disorientation, or general dementia. For those desiring a more comprehensive review of this topic, see Critchley[7] or Kinsbourne and Warrington.[25]

GERSTMANN SYNDROME

The Gerstmann syndrome is a classic, albeit controversial, neurologic syndrome. It consists of four major components: finger agnosia, right-left disorientation, dysgraphia, and dyscalculia. Most patients with this disorder, however, demonstrate additional neuropsychologic deficits, principally constructional impairment and mild aphasia. For specific details in evaluating the four major components of the Gerstmann syndrome, the reader is referred to the respective sections of this book (finger agnosia, p. 126; right-left disorientation, p. 125; dysgraphia, pp. 40, 46, 56; and dyscalculia, p. 116).

The syndrome has localizing value; the demonstration of all four elements indicates damage to the dominant parietal lobe.[31] The lesion is not necessarily restricted to the dominant hemisphere, however, since the Gerstmann syndrome is also frequently seen in patients with bilateral brain disease such as Alzheimer's disease or biparietal lesions. The reader desiring further information regarding this syndrome is referred to Benton,[4] Critchley,[9a] and Strub and Geschwind.[31]

VISUAL AGNOSIA

Visual agnosia is a rare, acquired neurologic syndrome in which the patient is unable to recognize objects or pictures of objects presented visually. Visual acuity is adequate, mentation clear, and aphasia absent.

Two major categories of visual agnosia have been described in the literature. In the first type, *actual visual perception* of the object is distorted to the point that recognition is impossible. Such patients are unable to name or tell the use of an object when it is shown to them, but can readily name and demonstrate the use of the object when it is placed in their hand. Kinesthetic cues provide sufficient information for recognition. To evaluate for the presence of visual agnosia, ask the patient to verbally identify common objects presented visually. If the patient fails to recognize the object, allow him to manipulate the object. If he readily identifies the object after manipulation, the defect is in the visual system. Finally, it is important to establish the adequacy of visual acuity. It has been postulated that such patients have damage to their visual association cortex bilaterally (areas 18 and 19). This type of visual agnosia has been reported in a patient with anoxic encephalopathy secondary to carbon dioxide poisoning.[3]

The second variety of visual agnosia is called *associative visual agnosia.* Patients with this type of agnosia have adequate visual perception, but have the visual cortex disconnected from the language area. Accordingly, they can recognize the object and demonstrate its use, but cannot name it. When unable to name an object, such patients are also unable to describe its use.[30] The evaluation for this disorder is similar to that for the first type of visual agnosia, except that adequate visual perception must be demonstrated. This can be done with a simple visual matching task. The lesion causing this associative agnosia is usually an infarct that destroys the left occipital lobe and the posterior corpus callosum.[26] This is the same lesion that causes alexia without agraphia (Chap. 4) and, in fact, most patients with associative visual agnosia are alexic. For further reading, refer to Critchley,[8] Bender and Feldman,[2] Lhermitte and Beauvois,[26] and Albert, Reches, and Silverberg.[1]

There are two additional types of visual agnosia which deserve mention, but will not be fully discussed. *Prosopagnosia* is an unusual agnosia in which patients are unable to recognize familiar faces. In such cases, the agnosia is so profound that even members of the patient's immediate family are not recognized. The patient will recognize the person, however, upon hearing his voice. The mechanism resulting in prosopagnosia is probably a combination of a disturbance of fine visual discrimination and a failure of memory for the discrete category of human faces. The lesions responsible for this disorder are usually in the occipitotemporal areas bilaterally. One of the lesions is usually in the right inferior temporo-occipital region.[27] For further references, see De Renzi and Spinnler,[14] Benton and Van Allen,[5] and Meadows.[27]

Color agnosia is an inability to recognize colors secondary to an acquired cortical lesion. Two types of color agnosia have been described. There is a specific color naming disturbance that results from a disconnection of visual input from the language area. This color anomia is associated with the syndrome of alexia with agraphia.[20] In this form there is no damage to the primary language area and no other evidence of aphasia.

The second and more common disturbance of color recognition is actually a defect in color perception caused by bilateral inferior temporo-occipital lesions. These are the same lesions that cause prosopagnosia and most patients with this type of color agnosia have concomitant prosopagnosia.[28] For further reading regarding this topic, refer to Critchley[9] and De Renzi et al.[12]

GEOGRAPHIC ORIENTATION

Geographic orientation is a complex ability which includes the patient's capacity to find his way in familiar environments, to localize places on maps or floor plans, and to find his way in new environments. A significant geographic disorientation will interfere with the patient's ability to live a normal life. Such patients are unable to travel alone outside their home and may even become disoriented within their own houses.

Evaluation

1. History Obtained from Family

In evaluating geographic orientation it is important to obtain historical information regarding the patient's ability to operate in familiar and unfamiliar environments outside the formal testing situation. Such information is best obtained from family members rather than from the patient himself.

a. Does the patient become lost at work, in his neighborhood, or at home?
b. Has he become lost traveling to a less frequented location (e.g., the inability to locate a restaurant that he had not been to in a year)?
c. Does he have great difficulty orienting to new environments?

2. Localizing Places on a Map

Map localization is an abstract task which can, however, quickly detect disturbances in geographic orientation. It is also useful when adequate historical information is unobtainable and may bring out subtle defects in unilateral attention.

Directions. Have the patient draw a map of the United States. If he is unable to produce a recognizable representation, the doctor should draw one or provide a suitable outline. Ask the patient to localize the following cities on the map outline.

1. Boston	4. Los Angeles
2. Seattle	5. New Orleans
3. Miami	6. Denver

Scoring. There are no well validated standards for scoring performance on this task. In reviewing the patient's performance, the following factors should be considered: (1) Are coastal cities located on the coast? (2) Are the cities in the appropriate states? (3) Are all cities in one half of the map (either east or west)? (4) Are attempts made to localize all cities?

Ability to Orient Self in Hospital Environment

Information concerning the patient's ability to orient himself in a new environment (hospital) may be obtained from nurses' reports and by observing the patient's capacity to find his bed, his ward, and the bathroom. For example, we recently saw a patient with communicating hydrocephalus and mild dementia who upon concluding a fifth office revisit, walked confidently into the closet.

Clinical Implications

Geographic disorientation has been clinically associated with parietal lobe disease,[7] though few good clinicoanatomic studies have been reported. Of the studies available, it is apparent that right hemisphere lesions most frequently cause geographic difficulty.[24] Other studies, however, have failed to support this finding of lateralization and report an approximately equal incidence of geographic disorientation in patients with right and left hemisphere lesions.[6]

A consistent finding of clinical utility is that patients with unilateral lesions tend to localize cities on the map toward the side of their lesion (e.g., patients with left parietal lesions tend to place cities toward the west coast on the map outline). This appears to be a result of neglect of the contralateral visual field.[6] A more generalized geographic disorientation is a frequent finding in patients with diffuse cortical disease and may be an early sign of dementing illness.

Geographic orientation is probably not a unitary cortical function, but a combination of more basic cognitive processes including visual memory, right-left orientation, visual perception, and spatial neglect. Performance on formal tests of geographic orientation such as locating cities on a map outline is closely associated with both general intelligence and social exposure (education).

One must not minimize the devastating effects that geographic disorientation has upon the patient's ability to function effectively in his environment. Such patients are typically unable to work, become easily lost in unfamiliar places, and eventually have difficulty with orientation in even familiar settings such as the neighborhood and home.

SUMMARY

The cortical functions of apraxia, visual and finger agnosia, geographic and right-left disorientation are interesting and may be clinically relevant in localizing brain lesions.

REFERENCES

1. Albert, M., Reches, A., and Silverberg, R.: Associative visual agnosia without alexia. Neurology 25:322, 1975.
2. Bender, M., and Feldman, M.: The so-called "visual agnosias." Brain 95:173, 1972.
3. Benson, F., and Greenberg, J.: Visual form agnosia. Arch. Neurol. 20:82, 1969.
4. Benton, A.: The fiction of the Gerstmann syndrome. J. Neurol. Neurosurg. Psychiatry 24:176, 1961.
5. Benton, A., and Van Allen, M.: Prosopagnosia and facial discrimination. J. Neurol. Sci. 15:167, 1972.
6. Benton, A., Levin, H., and Van Allen, M.: Geographic orientation in patients with unilateral cerebral disease. Neuropsychologia 12:183, 1974.
7. Critchley, M.: The Parietal Lobes. Edward Arnold & Company, London, 1953.
8. Critchley, M.: The problem of visual agnosia. J. Neurol. Sci. 1:274, 1964.
9. Critchley, M.: Acquired anomalies of colour perception of central origin. Brain 88:711, 1965.
9a. Critchley, M.: The enigma of Gerstmann's Syndrome. Brain 89:183, 1966.
10. De Ajuriagurerra, J., Hecaen, H., and Angelerques, R.: Les apraxies: Varietes cliniques et lateralisation lesionnelle. Rev. Neurol. 102:566, 1960.
11. Denny-Brown, D.: The nature of apraxia. J. Nerv. Ment. Dis. 126:9, 1958.

12. De Renzi, E., Faglioni, P., Scotti, G., and Spinnler, H.: Impairment in associating colour to form, concomitant with aphasia. Brain 95:293, 1972.
13. De Renzi, E., Pieczuro, A., and Vignolo, L.: Ideational apraxia: A quantitative study. Neuropsychologia 6:41, 1968.
14. De Renzi, E., and Spinnler, H.: Facial recognition in brain damaged patients. Neurology 16:145, 1966.
15. Frederiks, J.: Disorders of the body schema, in Vinken, P., and Bruyn, G. (eds.): Handbook of Clinical Neurology, Volume 4, Disorders of Speech, Perception and Symbolic Behavior. American Elsevier, New York, 1969, pp. 207–240.
16. Gerstmann, J.: Some notes on the Gerstmann-syndrome. Neurology 7:866, 1957.
17. Geschwind, N.: Sympathetic dyspraxia. Trans. Am. Neurol. Assoc. 88:219, 1963.
18. Geschwind, N.: Disconnection syndromes in animals and man. Part II. Brain 88:585, 1965.
19. Geschwind, N.: The apraxias: Neural mechanisms of disorders of learned movement. Am. Sci. 63:188, 1975.
20. Geschwind, N., and Fusillo, M.: Color-naming defects in association with alexia. Arch. Neurol. 15:137, 1966.
21. Geschwind, N., and Kaplan, E.: A human cerebral deconnection syndrome. Neurology 12:675, 1962.
22. Goodglass, H., and Kaplan, E.: The Assessment of Aphasia and Related Disorders. Lea and Febiger, Philadelphia, 1972.
23. Hecaen, H., and De Ajuriaguerra, J.: Meconnaissances et Hallucinations Corporelles. Masson et Cie. Paris, 1952.
24. Hecaen, H., and Angelerques, R.: La Cecite Psychique. Masson et Cie, Paris, 1963.
25. Kinsbourne, M., and Warrington, E.: A study of finger agnosia. Brain 85:47, 1962.
26. Lhermitte, F. and Beauvois, M.: A visual-speech disconnection syndrome. Brain 96:695, 1973.
27. Meadows, J.: The anatomical basis of prosopagnosia. J. Neurol. Neurosurg. Psychiatry 37:489, 1974.
28. Meadows, J.: Disturbed perception of colours associated with localized cerebral lesions. Brain 97:615, 1974.
29. Nielsen, J.: Gerstmann syndrome: Finger agnosia, agraphia, confusion of right and left, and acalculia. Arch. Neurol. Psychiatry 39:536, 1938.
30. Rubens, A., and Benson, D.: Associative visual agnosia. Arch. Neurol. 24:305, 1971.
31. Strub, R., and Geschwind, N.: Gerstmann syndrome without aphasia. Cortex 10:378, 1974.

CHAPTER 10

Summary of Examination

Throughout this book we have emphasized the importance of carrying out a systematic and complete mental status examination. Although it is not always necessary to exhaustively evaluate every aspect of mental functioning, there are certain critical functions which must be assessed in every patient. These include level of consciousness, appearance and emotional status, attention, expressive and receptive language (aphasia screening), memory, constructional ability, and abstract verbal reasoning. Items adequate for evaluating these areas are starred in the composite mental status examination (see Appendix 2). With practice, an adequate screening examination can be completed in 15 minutes.

The systematic mental status examination usually allows the clinician to accurately differentiate patients with organic brain disease from normal persons and those with functional disorders. In many cases it is also possible to specify the type, locus, and degree of disease. For example, knowledge of specific patterns of aphasia often permits the examiner to localize a lesion within the dominant hemisphere. In other cases, the pattern of performance is suggestive, if not pathognomonic, of a specific disease entity (i.e., Alzheimer's disease).

The usefulness of the mental status examination has been amply demonstrated both in the literature and in clinical practice. If, on the other hand, a mental status examination is not included in the routine neurologic evaluation, many patients with organic brain disease will be misdiagnosed. We have seen numerous patients with negative routine neurologic examinations who when evaluated with a systematic mental status examination demonstrated clear organic deficits which were subsequently documented by other neurodiagnostic procedures. Recently, a 51-year-old male under treatment in a psychiatric hospital for a depressive psychosis was referred for neurologic evaluation because of suspected papilledema. Although no papilledema was seen, the patient was apathetic and demonstrated significant difficulty with memory, calculations, right-left orientation, and abstract reasoning. These findings strongly suggested that the patient had Alzheimer's dementia and not a primary depression. A pneumoencephalogram documented cortical atrophy with marked dilatation of the sulci, increased basilar cisterns, and dilatation of the lateral and third ventricles. This type of atrophy is consistent with the diagnosis of Alzheimer's disease. Further examples of neurologic disease unrecognized because of the lack of systematic mental status examination are included in Geschwind.[1]

As with any medical examination it is very important to record both what was specifically tested and the patient's responses to each item. To aid in recording these data, forms similar to the composite mental status examination in Appendix 2 may be used. A systematic recording of data allows the clinician to accurately communicate his findings, document changes in the patient's status over time, and evaluate the effectiveness of any treatment. At the completion of the examination, the clinician should synthesize the data and then summarize and emphasize the key areas of impairment. This summary allows an identification of patterns of deficit and the efficient communication of essential findings.

In the Clinical Implications sections of each chapter in this book, we have attempted to describe many neurobehavioral syndromes as they relate to specific areas of cognitive deficit. Examples of this are the acute confusional states (Chap. 3), aphasias and related language disorders (Chap. 5), amnesias (Chap. 6), and the frontal lobe syndrome (Chap. 3). A description of several common patterns of cognitive impairment illustrating how findings from the mental status examination can lead to a neurologic diagnosis appear below. This section is not intended as a comprehensive review of neurobehavior nor as an intensive discussion of any one syndrome. It is, rather, an illustration of the bridge between the data and the diagnosis.

DOMINANT HEMISPHERE LESIONS

Patients with lesions of the dominant hemisphere will frequently show abnormalities of language functions. In the right handed patient, evidence of aphasia, alexia, or agraphia almost always indicates left hemisphere disease. The Gerstmann syndrome, constructional impairment, verbal memory difficulties, ideomotor apraxia, dyscalculia, and impairment of verbal reasoning are all findings that can be seen with left hemisphere lesions. Denial and neglect are not commonly seen in these patients. Even left handed patients will frequently show the above findings with left hemisphere disease, although there is a higher frequency of bilateral representation of the above functions in these patients.

NONDOMINANT HEMISPHERE LESIONS

Most patients with lesions of the nondominant hemisphere will not show evidence of language disorders. They do have a more dramatic constructional impairment than patients with dominant hemisphere lesions. Denial and neglect are more common and severe in degree, malalignment is seen in writing and calculations, and deficits are present in nonverbal memory.

ALZHEIMER'S DISEASE/SENILE DEMENTIA

Alzheimer's disease is by far the most common of the dementing illnesses and one seen routinely by every clinician. It is important to recognize the early features of this syndrome as early diagnosis can prevent serious social and vocational embarrassment to the patient and his family (see Chap. 11). The early features of this disease which can readily be demonstrated on a systematic mental status examination are apathy, vague subjective complaints, memory difficulties, constructional impairment, and problems with abstract reasoning. As the disease progresses, anomia, apraxia, agnosia, geographic disorientation, and significant deficits in judgment typically appear. There is also a worsening of those defects seen in the early stages of the disease. In the deteriorated stage, all deficits are accentuated, behavior is regressed, language, memory, and thought processes are severely disturbed, and the patients require total care. The diagnosis of Alzheimer's disease in the advanced stages is usually made without difficulty. However, it is surprising how often mild, but significant dementia goes unrecognized by family and physician alike.

Traditionally, Alzheimer's disease has been considered a devastating presenile dementia that leads to total helplessness and death within a few years of onset. The term senile dementia on the other hand was applied to cases of dementia that began after the age of 60 and had a slower less dramatic course with less extensive pathologic changes. This differentiation has proven artificial since cases fitting the classic Alzheimer's pattern can occur at any age and the clinical and pathologic features of both conditions are identical.[3] For a recent review of this problem, see Katzman.[2]

These examples demonstrate the application of mental status examination findings in describing cognitive and emotional deficits, deriving tentative neurobehavioral and clinical diagnoses, and establishing a localization of the lesion when possible. Data necessary for arriving at these conclusions can usually be obtained by the experienced examiner in 15 to 20 minutes. The clinician unfamiliar with mental status testing will want to devote additional time understanding all aspects of the complete examination and applying it to a variety of patients. With experience each examiner will develop a comfortable examination routine that he can readily apply at the bedside or in the office.

The final steps in any patient evaluation include communicating test findings to the patient, his family, and the referring physician; referring for further evaluation when necessary; and arranging for appropriate subsequent patient management.

REFERENCES

1. Geschwind, N.: The borderland of neurology and psychiatry: Some common misconceptions, in Benson, D. F., and Blumer, D. (eds.): Psychiatric Aspects of Neurological Disease. Grune and Stratton, New York, 1975, pp. 1-8.
2. Katzman, R.: The prevalence and malignancy of Alzheimer disease. Arch. Neurol. 33:217, 1976.
3. Katzman, R., and Karasu, T.: Differential diagnosis of dementia, in Fields, W. (ed.): Neurological and Sensory Disorders in the Elderly. Stratton Intercontinental Medical Book Corp., New York, 1975, pp. 103-134.

CHAPTER 11

Further Evaluations

After completion of the routine mental status examination, there are a number of situations in which additional more comprehensive evaluation of specific aspects of performance is warranted. This section will briefly discuss the contributions of the neuropsychologist, speech pathologist, and psychiatrist in the total evaluation of the patient with organic brain disease.

NEUROPSYCHOLOGY

The clinical neuropsychologist is trained at the Ph.D. level in a four to five year academic program with a one year clinical internship in which practice is given in the use of standard psychologic tests and specialized neuropsychologic techniques to evaluate patients with organic brain disease. Their training generally includes neuroanatomy, physiology, and rudimentary clinical neurology in addition to the topics of a more traditional psychologic nature. The clinical neuropsychologist is primarily concerned with the identification, quantification, and description of changes in behavior which are associated with brain dysfunction. By reason of his specialized training, the clinical neuropsychologist's area of interest and expertise is the relationships between human behavior (whether specific to a response on a formal test or in general) and brain function. Accordingly, his activities can contribute to a variety of important clinical problems including differential diagnosis, lateralization and localization of lesions, establishment of baselines of behavior and cognitive performance from which improvement or deterioration can be gauged, determination of competency in the aged or demented, and development of remedial methods for the rehabilitation of the individual brain damaged patient.[9]

The neuropsychologic evaluation briefly defined is an objective comprehensive assessment of a wide range of cognitive, adaptive, and emotional behaviors which reflect the adequacy (or inadequacy) of cortical functioning. In essence, the neuropsychologic evaluation is a greatly expanded and objectified mental status examination. The mental status examination is designed to briefly (15 to 30 minutes) screen a variety of critical areas, while the neuropsychologic evaluation assesses a wider range of performance in more depth over a longer period of time (2 to 6 hours). It differs from the mental status examination in that it generally uses tests and evaluation procedures which have been standardized with samples of either normals (e.g., Wechsler series of intelligence scales) or brain damaged patients (e.g., Memory for Designs Test or the Trail Making Test). Because of this use of standardized measures, comparisons can be made of the individual patient's performance with that of standard groups as well as the varying adequacy of the same patient's performance across a variety of test areas. The objective and highly quantified nature of most neuropsychologic tests aids in the detection of subtle changes in performance over time (e.g., the slowly deteriorating dementia or the improvement in specific functions after neurosurgery). Because of the wide range of performance assessed and the depth in which it is evaluated, the neuropsychologic evaluation may detect subtle deficits not apparent on the mental status examination.

The neuropsychologic evaluation has a number of advantages not shared by many standard neurodiagnostic techniques. It is noninvasive and has no risk of mortality or morbidity; these factors make the evaluation appropriate for patients for whom the risk of invasive procedures (pneumoencephalography or angiography) is too great or for whom the probability of positive findings is sufficiently small that any risk is too high (e.g., the child with soft neurologic signs of "minimal brain dysfunction" on general clinical exam). The neuropsychologic tests are interesting to most patients and do not produce the potential complications of anxiety and pain of some invasive procedures. The evaluation also provides important descriptive and prognostic information that other techniques cannot. This is especially true in regard to a description of the effects of neurologic disease upon the patient as a person and its probable impact upon academic, social, and vocational adjustment.

The physician without ready access to a trained neuropsychologist may, nonetheless, benefit from evaluation performed by clinical psychologists who have had some experience in evaluating patients with brain damage. This is especially true if the referring physician is familiar with the types of data provided by the psychologist and knows how to interpret the reports. A review of the information contained in this section and in the appendix of psychologic tests should greatly aid in this interpretation.

A common feature of the psychologic reports provided by persons other than neuropsychologists which may be difficult to interpret without some knowledge of its meaning is the frequent reporting of so-called "organic signs." Such signs typically include the following:

1. Verbal-performance discrepancies, i.e., appreciable differences between the Verbal and Performance Scale IQs on the Wechsler series of intelligence tests. Differences exceeding 25 points are statistically significant,[4] while differences of 15 points have been shown to be of some clinical utility in identifying neurologic dysfunction.[1] Reported verbal-performance discrepancies must be cautiously interpreted in the light of the overall psychologic test profile and of any primary sensory or motor deficit (e.g., a visual impairment or cerebral palsy).

2. A scattering of performance levels on the various subtests of the Wechsler tests or among any scores obtained from the full psychologic test battery (e.g., a subtest score of 12 on the WAIS Vocabulary Subtest and 6 on the Similarities Subtest). Such differential performance does indicate discrepant intellectual functioning which should be explained. The physician should recognize, however, that a number of factors (social, psychologic, and educational) other than brain damage may result in such subtest "scatter." Accordingly, this sign should not be interpreted in isolation as indicating brain damage.

3. An indication of visual motor dysfunction as detected by any measure of constructional ability, including the nonverbal WAIS subtests, the Bender Gestalt, drawings to command, etc. The best predictors of brain damage are specific errors of rotation and perseveration. Errors related to the integration of parts or the distortion of the gestalt tend to be maturational rather than pathologic. Constructional ability and its impairment is covered in depth in Chapter 7. Suffice to say, a wide variety of social, maturational, motor, and sensory factors as well as brain damage may impinge upon constructional ability, so information regarding performance in this area must be evaluated within the context of the total psychologic evaluation and the patient's history.

4. Behavioral findings include hyperactivity, distractability, mixed dominance, motor incoordination, clumsiness, and so forth. It is well established that the incidence of such behaviors is higher in brain damaged individuals than in normals, especially among children. The use of such behavioral indicators in isolation as diagnostic of brain damage is, however, unwarranted in light of present knowledge.

In sum, the information provided by the clinical psychologist may be of significant value to the physician in describing the abilities and disabilities of the patient and in helping to make a diagnosis of brain damage. The referring physician must, however, utilize the services of a well trained and experienced psychologist, understand something of the nature of the commonly employed psychologic tests, and be able to interpret both the utility and the limitations of the so-called brain damage indicators or "organic signs."

Referral

Appropriate referrals for neuropsychologic evaluation are comprised of patients for whom the physician requires further information in regards to diagnosis, description of the effects of a well verified lesion upon behavior, and prognosis and management.

Cognitive and behavioral disturbances may occur in the absence of any clear-cut physical signs of cerebral disease on standard clinical neurologic exam; this is particularly true in cases of early dementia. Dementia typically presents with vague behavioral complaints such as mental dullness, concentration problems, increasing apathy and loss of interest in job or family, chronic fatigue without apparent organic etiology, depression, and memory problems. The neuropsychologic evaluation of such patients can often contribute to an early diagnosis. The common diagnostic problem of differentiating between dementia and depression is frequently solved by the data obtained in the neuropsychologic battery. The neuropsychologic evaluation may also provide supporting data for the diagnosis of brain dysfunction and serve as a basis for ordering more extensive and specific neurodiagnostic procedures.

The evaluation can also determine the relative impact of the organic and functional components in a patient with both neurologic and psychiatric complaints.

Any patient with a brain lesion should receive a neuropsychologic evaluation as part of his rehabilitation program. The comprehensive nature of the evaluation can provide valuable information regarding the effect of the lesion upon cognitive functioning, emotional status, behavior, and social adjustment. Objective data will elucidate both specific areas of impairment and residual abilities. This outline of strengths and weaknesses is valuable in describing the effects of specific neurologic lesions upon the individual patient and provides information critical for vocational and social rehabilitation.

Serial testing can provide reliable objective information regarding the speed and degree of recovery after brain injury or after neurosurgical procedures. Similarly, repeated evaluations can be used to assess deterioration in cases of progressive disease or to rule out such progression in equivocal cases. Preneurosurgical and postneurosurgical evaluation may help to quantify the effects of surgery upon the cognitive, behavioral, vocational, and social functioning of the patient. In a similar sense, the effects of any medical treatment (e.g., levodopa in Parkinsonism or anticonvulsants in epilepsy) may be well documented by pretreatment and posttreatment neuropsychologic evaluation. These changes over time are difficult to assess without an adequate baseline of data encompassing a wide range of cognitive functions and behavior.

It is apparent that in any case of trauma or suspected brain damage involving litigation or compensation, the objective data obtained from neuropsychologic evaluation are of great value in documenting and describing the presence, absence, or degree of disability. There is considerable legal precedence for the admission of testimony of psychologists as expert witnesses.

The Neuropsychologic Evaluation

Below is a summary of the clinical services which can be provided by the neuropsychologist.

Categorization. This section provides information as to the presence or absence of brain dysfunction and the presence or absence of significant emotional disturbance. The differential diagnosis of a primary organic or a primary functional disorder is made. If significant components of both organic and functional features are present, the relative impact of the two will be discussed.

Localization. Typically, performance on the neuropsychologic test battery can be analyzed to provide data to determine if the brain dysfunction is diffuse or focal. Further analysis provides data as to the lateralization of the lesion in the right or left hemisphere and localization of the lesion in the anterior or posterior regions of the hemisphere.

Description. Information included in this category pertains to a comprehensive description of the patient's current level of functioning in a wide range of cognitive, adaptive, personality, and behavioral areas. From the academic and social history and an analysis of the variability of performance on various tests, it is generally possible to make an estimate of the patient's premorbid level of functioning. From comparisons of the estimated premorbid level of functioning and current performance on standard tests, an accurate indication of deterioration in any of the areas assessed by the battery may be made. A comprehensive overview of the patient's deficits and residual abilities is made to provide a description of current functioning, explain present behavior, determine the relative effects of organic and functional factors, and provide a baseline of data from which to judge future change. Documented statements should be made to help the primary physician determine the effect of the patient's neurologic disease and its associated deficits upon his subsequent academic, vocational, and social adjustment. Answers to the question of mental competency and social independence can also be provided by data obtained in the neuropsychologic evaluation.

Prognosis and Recommendations. Based upon the nature of the neurologic disease and the pattern and degree of deficits seen during neuropsychologic evaluation, a determination of the probability and degree of expected recovery can be made for many patients. As previously mentioned, serial evaluations some months apart aid greatly in the ability to make valid prognostic statements in case of either deterioration or recovery. Finally, recommendations for further ancillary evaluations including psychiatric, speech pathology, occupational therapy, and social service are made when warranted. Recommendations regarding specific remedial methods or programs may also be made.

Components of the Neuropsychologic Evaluation. Specific tests employed in a neuropsychologic evaluation battery will vary with the age of the patient and the nature of the problems, specific referral questions asked by the referring physician, and the particular training and experience of the psychologist. Virtually all such test batteries will, however, include objective tests of the following functions:

1. Behavior, attention, and mood
2. Intelligence, including general intelligence, verbal intelligence, and nonverbal intelligence
3. Language, including single word and sentence comprehension, auditory discrimination, and various aspects of expressive language
4. Memory, including verbal and nonverbal memory, short and long term memory, and new learning ability
5. Abstract ability, including verbal and nonverbal abstract reasoning
6. Constructional ability, including paper and pencil reproductions, construction, and reproduction from memory
7. Geographic orientation
8. Temporal orientation
9. Achievement, including reading, spelling, and calculations
10. Perceptual motor speed, including the ability to plan ahead and shift concepts rapidly
11. Motor strength and coordination
12. Personality

References to specific tests tapping these functions may be seen in Appendix 1.

In sum, we have found that neurologists and neuropsychologists can beneficially work closely together and make mutually rewarding contributions in the evaluation, description, and management of patients with cognitive and behavioral changes secondary to organic brain disease.

Those wishing further, more detailed information regarding neuropsychologic testing are recommended to review Reitan and Davidson,[11] Russell, Neuringer, and Goldstein,[12] Small,[14] or Smith and Philippus.[15]

SPEECH PATHOLOGY

Patients with significant difficulty communicating should be evaluated by a trained speech pathologist. All such patients will not be treatment candidates, but by means of the thorough language evaluation, the speech pathologist is best able to determine appropriate candidates for rehabilitation and provide other services to patients not selected for treatment. Patients with aphasia, apraxia of speech, or dysarthria are examples of primary neurologic patients that are appropriate for referral. The speech pathologist should be an important member of any comprehensive rehabilitation team; this is particularly true when a unit sees a large number of stroke patients. Functional speech and language disorders such as elective mutism and hysterical aphonia are ideal conditions for speech evaluation and treatment. Evaluation by the speech pathologist provides a description of the patient's level of communication, the possible benefits of therapeutic intervention, and a plan for family counseling to facilitate alternate methods of communicating with the patient.

Virtually every physician has access to speech pathologists either in private practice or in hospital, university, or community clinics. The speech pathologist may be trained at either the master's or doctoral level; most clinicians will hold the master's degree. The American Speech and Hearing Association and many states issue licenses or certificates of clinical competence to qualified clinicians. The referring physician should ensure the basic clinical competence of any speech pathologist he consults. Many speech pathologists will have specialized knowledge and experience in treating patients with delayed speech acquisition, articulation disorders, stuttering, or aphasia. The evaluation and treatment of aphasia is a very specialized field and the physician should determine the speech pathologist's competence in this area before referring his aphasic patients.

Referral

The major reasons for referring patients to the speech pathologist are:

1. The mental status indicates a communication disorder that requires a more thorough evaluation.

2. Obvious communication disorders that require a screening evaluation to determine the appropriateness of speech therapy.

3. The significant communication disorder that requires family counseling to inform the family members as to the patient's problem and to assist in maximizing communication in the home.

The physician will see the following general types of speech and language problems which will require more comprehensive evaluation than can be provided in the office:

1. Articulation disturbances such as the dysarthrias as seen in pseudobulbar palsy, bulbar paralysis, neuromuscular disease such as myasthenia

gravis, cerebellar disorders, cerebral palsy, and basal ganglia disease such as Parkinsonism.

2. Functional (hysterical) aphonias, especially in patients with histories of minor trauma or surgery to the throat or vocal cords.

3. Elective mutism.

4. Dysfluency (stuttering). This disorder is seen in both children and adults and, if untreated, may pose a significant obstacle to successful social and vocational adjustment.

5. Patients with acquired language disorders (aphasia, alexia, agraphia) deserve an initial speech and language evaluation, both to determine the potential for speech therapy and to aid the patient's family in understanding and dealing with the communication disorder. Because of the rapid changes in language which occur during the first two to four weeks following an acute cerebral lesion, speech evaluations will be most valid and prognostically useful if carried out after this initial period.

6. Patients with buccofacial apraxia in the presence or absence of aphasia may benefit from speech evaluation and therapy directed toward articulation and the intelligibility of speech, as well as other buccofacial activities such as drinking and swallowing.

7. The childhood developmental disorders of speech delay, reading and writing disabilities, and other specific learning disorders. It is critical that the child with such developmental disabilities receive a comprehensive evaluation and treatment program. At least the evaluation component of the program would include input from speech pathology.

Speech and Language Evaluation

The comprehensive speech and language evaluation can be expected to provide information regarding:

Diagnosis. A definition of the primary language diagnosis (e.g., nonfluent aphasia, dysarthria, buccofacial apraxia, etc.).

Description. A comprehensive description of the type of language disorder, including all areas of deficit (e.g., word finding problems, alexia, or auditory comprehension problems) and residual language abilities. The description should contain some qualitative index of the degree of problem in each area assessed to allow comparison with subsequent evaluations. Some statement should be made as to the effect of the language deficit upon the patient's communicative ability in formal (test or interview) and information (social) areas.

Recommendations. Is speech therapy indicated and if so what will be the emphasis of the therapy? What will be the frequency of therapy visits, what is the projected duration of therapy, and what are the specific plans for home therapy by family members and for family counseling?

Goals of Therapy and Prognosis. What are the primary goals of speech and language therapy? What is the prognosis for language recovery? What will be the long term social impact of the language disorder?

Components of the Speech and Language Evaluation. There are numerous systems and methods of speech and language evaluation. The system and specific tests employed will be determined in part by the particular patient and partly by the individual speech pathologist's training and experience. As the enumeration of these methods is beyond the scope of this book, the interested reader is referred to the following texts and manuals Eisenson,[3] Goodglass and Kaplan,[5] Porch,[10] Schuell.[13]

A comprehensive evaluation should include the following elements:

1. An examination of the oral physiology, to include the strength and alacrity of the muscles of articulation.

2. A description of the characteristics of speech articulation—dysarthria, dysfluency, and dysprosody.

3. A description of apraxias if present, both verbal (speech) and nonverbal (nonspeech facial movements).

4. An evaluation for aphasia, to specifically include an assessment of verbal comprehension, repetition, and word finding ability, and a description of spontaneous speech.

5. An assessment of reading and writing.

6. An evaluation of the adequacy of nonverbal communication, to include an assessment of the ability to communicate utilizing gestures or other methods regardless of the language deficit.

7. A description of the patient's general behavior and specific behavioral responses to the stress of language items.

Treatment

Treatment is not universally efficacious in all speech and language disorders. The following is a general breakdown of the expected results with a number of patient types based upon our clinical experience.

Excellent results can often be produced in rehabilitating patients with (1) functional voice disorders, exclusive of elective mutism (which is more resistant to traditional forms of speech therapy), (2) mild to moderate articulation problems, and (3) nonretarded children with delayed speech.

Good results can be expected in patients with (1) anomic aphasia, (2) oral apraxia, (3) moderate articulation problems, and (4) developmental reading and learning disorders.

Fair results are generally obtained in patients with (1) Broca's aphasia, (2) moderate to severe articulation problems, (3) aphasia with mild to moderate comprehension defects, (4) developmental aphasia, and (5) elective mutism (unless intensive behaviorally oriented therapy is employed in which case the prognosis is improved).

Poor results are typical in therapeutic efforts with patients with (1) global aphasia, (2) Wernicke's aphasia, (3) severe dysarthria and oral apraxia, and (4) language disturbances secondary to dementia.

It is emphasized that this is a general classification scheme; the individual patient with a particular language disorder will not always respond to therapy as projected. Accordingly, a speech and language evaluation of the patient with any developmental or acquired communication disorder is important to provide the opportunity for therapy to patients who may benefit from it.

PSYCHIATRY

Many patients with organic brain disease will have concomitant emotional disturbance which requires psychiatric consultation. Patients referred for psychiatric evaluation include those with psychiatric disorders preceding their neurologic problem, those with emotional reactions to brain disease (e.g., reactive depression), patients in whom an emotional reaction complicates dementia, and those with functional disorders presenting as neurologic conditions (e.g., hysterical paralysis).

Emotional factors are significant in the rehabilitation and social reintegration of any patient with organic disease and the psychiatrist should be consulted to aid in the management of any patient with an emotional disturbance sufficiently severe to interfere with rehabilitative efforts or home adjustment.

Referral

Because of the relatively high incidence of both mental illness and brain disease, many patients will have coexisting psychiatric and neurologic conditions (e.g., a brain tumor in a schizophrenic patient or a seizure patient with a manic-depressive disorder). As a specific example, we recently saw a 37-year-old woman with a 7 year history of schizophrenia. The patient was also an alcoholic and over the years has sustained several significant head injuries. After alcohol withdrawal, she had several grand mal seizures and was admitted to the neurology ward. As her postictal confusion cleared, she demonstrated gross delusional and aggressive behavior. After a complete history and medical evaluation, we determined that the patient had an acute neurologic condition superimposed upon a pre-existing schizophrenia. Because of the significant functional psychosis, psychiatry was consulted for treatment and long term management. In general, psychiatrists should be consulted on patients with pre-existing psychiatric disease regardless of the nature of the coexisting medical disorder.

It is not uncommon for emotionally stable individuals to develop a significant emotional reaction to a recent neurobehavioral disorder such as aphasia. Depressive reactions, anxiety, paranoia, and aggressiveness may all develop in response to brain damage. Such emotional reactions may significantly interefere with rehabilitation efforts. As an example, a 62-year-old woman developed a right hemiplegia and anomic aphasia secondary to a cerebral thrombosis. After the acute stage, she became increasingly depressed to a point of apathy, self-depreciation, and constant crying. She would no longer actively participate in physical therapy and appeared to abandon any hope of improvement. When a serious emotional reaction such as this is superimposed on an organic deficit, the emotional component must be treated in conjunction with medical treatment. Psychiatric referral in the course of such cases will aid the total rehabilitation program.

Demented patients present a particular challenge because they have both intellectual and emotional changes as a part of their disease. These changes produce a variety of difficult management problems which are often best handled with the aid of a psychiatrist. In the early stage of dementia patients may retain considerable insight; this capacity to realize the seriousness of their condition often results in profound depression. Other dementing patients become unaware of their deteriorating intellectual ability; such patients often push themselves beyond their capability and develop frustration and severe anxiety. This situation was aptly illustrated by a recent case: A 58-year-old businessman was referred because of failing memory. His examination revealed a genuine memory deficit and other evidence of an early dementia. Severe anxiety was prominent and interferred with both specific test performance and his social and vocational life. This anxiety was greatly reduced by restructuring his lifestyle (e.g., his wife helped him with his business, he discontinued many civic duties, and used a mild tranquilizer to sleep). After several months, retesting showed improvement in many cognitive areas and he was better able to carry out his home and job responsibilities. Any anxiety or depression can greatly exacerbate any mental and social disability experienced by the demented patient. The psychiatrist can provide great assistance through the use of psychotrophic drugs, family counseling, and general patient management.

The diagnostic problem of differentiating among dementia, depression, and dementia with depression is both common and difficult in clinical practice. Because this differential diagnosis is critical in terms of patient management and treatment, the psychiatrist should be involved early in the evaluation process. The misdiagnosis of depression as dementia will deprive the patient of appropriate treatment and leave the family with the erroneous impression that the disease is progressive and irreversible. Conversely, the misdiagnosis of dementia as depression may lead to ineffective and costly psychotherapy, leaves the patient subject to the social and vocational problems resulting from intellectual deterioration, and misleads the family as to the prognosis of the disease.

Psychiatric referral is also indicated for patients who develop depression in response to a chronic neurologic disease such as myasthenia gravis, epilepsy, multiple sclerosis, or Parkinsonism. These patients frequently live long and productive lives if they are able to accept and deal with their disability in a realistic fashion.

Many patients with chronic organic brain syndromes like aphasia, dementia, traumatic encephalopathy, or Korsakoff's disease become management problems and eventually require long term care in a psychiatric hospital. Early referral to the psychiatrist or psychiatric social worker can help the family and the physician with the administrative and legal details involved in institutionalization.

A final group of patients who may initially be seen by the neurologist, but require referral to the psychiatrist, are the hysterical conversion reactions. Many patients will present with symptoms which mimic neurologic disease (e.g., limb paralysis, loss of speech, or sensory loss), but which demonstrate no organic etiology. The treatment of such functional disorders is psychotherapy.

Evaluation

The psychiatrist utilizes psychiatric interview techniques, a psychiatrically oriented mental status examination, and personality tests in his evaluation. Information on specific interview and evaluation techniques is readily available in all major psychiatric texts.[2,6,7,8,16]

Treatment

Even though specific treatment is frequently unavailable for the primary brain disease, behavioral and pharamacologic treatment can often improve the lives of most of these patients.

Medication is particularly useful in patients with pre-existing psychiatric disease. In such patients, the underlying psychiatric disorder will respond to a standard regimen of psychotrophic medication. Antianxiety or mood elevating drugs are effective in treating the anxiety or depression frequently seen as a reaction to organic brain disease. Major tranquilizers are often required to control the agitation and nocturnal wanderings of the deteriorated organic patient.

Standard psychotherapeutic methods can be used in some organic patients who retain comprehension, memory, and insight. On the other hand, insight therapy would be useless in many patients (e.g., severe amnesics, demented patients, those with significant frontal lobe behavioral changes, and Wernicke's aphasics). In this latter group of patients, behavior modification techniques to change specific behaviors are more appropriate and successful.

Family counseling is often the most useful form of patient management. Through discussion, the psychiatrist is able to help the family understand the patient's problem and to offer suggestions on management. With the psychiatrist's help, the family can then restructure the patient's routine in an effort to minimize environmental stress.

The medical-legal aspects of organic disease are also very important and must be part of a long term management program. The patient's competence to make a will, to conduct personal financial affairs, and to enter into contracts such as marriage should be established in each case.

Finally, every treatment plan should include a consideration of possible eventual full time supervision if the patient becomes unmanageable in the home. The details of nursing home or institutional placement should be worked out with the help of the psychiatrist, social worker, and the patient's family. Such plans should be considered early in the course to allow time to assess family financial and personal resources; to determine the availability of home nursing services, nursing homes, and institutions; and to preclude the necessity of unsatisfactory and hasty decisions made at a time of crisis.

SUMMARY

The management of patients with organic brain disease is a multidisciplinary effort. Physicians are strongly encouraged to acquaint themselves with the services offered by their colleagues in related specialized fields. With this effort, the physician will be able to better understand his patients and to provide them more comprehensive care.

REFERENCES

1. Black, W.: WISC verbal-performance discrepancies as indicators of neurological dysfunction in pediatric patients. J. Clin. Psychol. 30:165, 1974.
2. Detre, T., and Kupfer, D.: Psychiatric history and mental status examination, in Freedman, A., Kaplan, H., and Sadock, B. (eds.): Comprehensive Psychiatry. Williams & Wilkins, Baltimore, 1975, pp. 724–736.
3. Eisenson, J.: Examining for Aphasia. The Psychological Corporation, New York, 1954.
4. Field, J.: Two types of tables for use with Wechsler's intelligence scales. J. Clin. Psychol. 16:3, 1960.
5. Goodglass, H., and Kaplan, E.: The Assessment of Aphasia and Related Disorders. Lea & Febiger, Philadelphia, 1972.

149

6. Gregory, I.: Psychiatric interviewing and evaluation, in Fundamentals of Psychiatry. W. B. Saunders, Philadelphia, 1968, pp. 192-207.
7. Kolb, L.: Noyes's Modern Clinical Psychiatry. W. B. Saunders, Philadelphia, 1968, pp. 147-158.
8. Novello, J.: The psychiatric history and mental status examination, in Novello, J. (ed.): A Practical Handbook of Psychiatry. Charles C Thomas, Springfield, Ill., 1974, pp. 40-48.
9. Parsons, O: Clinical neuropsychology, in Speilberger, C. (ed.): Current Topics in Clinical and Community Psychology, Vol. 2. Academic Press, New York, 1970, pp. 1-60.
10. Porch, B.: Porch Index of Communicative Ability. Consulting Psychologists Press, Palo Alto, 1967.
11. Reitan, R., and Davidson, L. (eds.): Clinical Neuropsychology: Current Status and Applications. John Wiley & Sons, New York, 1974.
12. Russell, E., Neuringer, C., and Goldstein, G.: Assessment of Brain Damage. Wiley-Interscience, New York, 1970.
13. Schuell, H.: Differential Diagnosis of Aphasia with the Minnesota Test. University of Minnesota Press, Minneapolis, 1965.
14. Small, L.: Neuropsychodiagnosis in Psychotherapy. Brunner/Mazel, New York, 1973.
15. Smith, L., and Philippus, M. (eds.): Neuropsychological Testing in Organic Brain Dysfunction. Charles C Thomas, Springfield, Ill., 1969.
16. Stevenson, I., and Sheppe, W.: The psychiatric examination, in Arieti, S. (ed.): The American Handbook of Psychiatry, Vol. 1. Basic Books, New York, 1959, pp. 215-234.

APPENDIX 1

Standard Psychologic Tests

The following section provides a brief introduction to a number of commonly used standard psychologic tests which are used to assess brain damaged patients. It is not intended as a comprehensive review of all neuropsychologic procedures nor as an intensive evaluation of any individual technique. The purpose is to familiarize the interested reader with tests often mentioned in psychologic evaluation reports. A number of these tests can be readily adapted for inclusion in a more comprehensive office evaluation of patients with neurologic disease. Several tests mentioned are excellent screening instruments when used with the routine mental status examination.

Letters in parentheses following test names refer to the following publishers and test distributors:

A. American Guidance Services, Inc.
   Publishers' Building
   Circle Pines, Minnesota 55014
B. Charles C Thomas
   301-327 East Lawrence Avenue
   Springfield, Illinois 62717
C. Consulting Psychologists Press
   577 College Avenue
   Palo Alto, California 94806
D. Lea & Febiger
   600 Washington Square
   Philadelphia, Pennsylvania 19106
E. Neuropsychology Laboratory
   7708 89th Place, S.E.
   Mercer Island, Washington 98040
F. Neuropsychology Laboratory
   University of Victoria
   Victoria, British Columbia CANADA

G. The Psychological Corporation
   304 East 45th Street
   New York, New York 10017
H. Psychological Test Specialists
   Box 1441
   Missoula, Montana 59801
I. Western Psychological Services
   12031 Wilshire Blvd.
   Los Angeles, California 90025

COMPREHENSIVE NEUROPSYCHOLOGIC BATTERY

Halstead-Reitan Battery (E)

This battery, which is indeed comprehensive, includes a series of tests of cognitive and adaptive ability originally introduced by Halstead,[15] revised and standardized by Reitan and his coworkers,[25,30] and statistically refined by Russell et al.[32] The battery includes tests of verbal and non-verbal intelligence, concept formation, expressive and receptive language, auditory perception, time perception, memory, perceptual motor speed, tactile performance, spatial relations, finger gnosis, and double simultaneous stimulation. It is probably the best standardized and most widely reported neuropsychologic test battery in use in the United States at this time. The primary drawbacks of this battery are those of time and economy; the testing requires five to ten hours of trained examiner time and interpretation of the test results requires a highly trained clinical neuropsychologist.

INTELLIGENCE

Kent Series of Emergency Scales (G)

The Emergency Scales are comprised of a short series of simple verbal questions which provides a rapid screening estimate of general intellectual functioning. The advantages of the test are its ease and speed of administration and interpretation (five minutes), while its disadvantages are related to its brevity and the lack of adequate reliability and validity data.[19]

Progressive Matrices Test (G, I)

The test is a series of progressively more difficult matrices which provides an assessment of nonverbal intelligence in a relatively brief time. Responses can be made either verbally or nonverbally, making the test useful for use with patients with language or motor deficits. The test has also been used as a measure of right hemisphere function by some researchers.[6,24]

The Quick Test (H)

This is a picture vocabulary test of intelligence which may be useful as a rapid screening measure when time is at a premium. The test involves a verbal administration and a nonverbal pointing response. As with most screening tests of intelligence, the Quick Test suffers from a lack of standardization and adequate research support of its validity and reliability. It is not intended as a substitute for a more comprehensive test of intelligence.[1]

Wechsler Adult Intelligence Scale (G)

The WAIS is the 1955 revision and restandardization of the Wechsler-Bellvue Scale. It is a well constructed and standardized test which is generally recognized as the standard measure of intelligence when time (1 to 1.5 hours) allows its use. The test evaluates performance in six verbal areas: social information (e.g., What is the capitol of Italy?), comprehension (e.g., Why should people pay taxes?), arithmetic (e.g., A man with $18 spends $7.50. How much does he have left?), similarities (e.g., In what way are air and water alike?), vocabulary (i.e., verbal definitions), and digit repetition both forward and backward. It also tests nonverbal performance in the areas of digit symbol (written symbol coding), block design constructions reproduced from a pictorial stimulus, picture arrangement (visual sequencing of a series of pictures which complete a story), picture completion (recognition of omitted details from pictured objects), and object assembly (construction of picture puzzles). The discrepancy between Verbal and Performance Scale IQs and the variations among subtest scores may be used to determine specific areas of strength and weakness and, with some caution, to aid in cerebral localization. Clinical use of the test requires specialized training and experience in both its administration and interprettion.[21,38]

MEMORY

Wechsler Memory Scale (G)

This is a relatively brief (30 minutes) memory battery for clinical use. The WMS assesses the areas of personal and current information (e.g., In what year were you born? Who is the governor of your state?), orientation to time and place (e.g., What is the month? What is the name of this place?), mental control (tested by counting backwards from 20 to 1, reciting the alphabet, and counting by serial 3s), logical memory (i.e., the immediate recall of a paragraph read aloud by the examiner), digit repetition both forward and backward, visual memory (i.e., paper and pencil reproduction of simple designs from memory), and paired associate learning (using pairs with strong natural associations—baby and cries—and pairs without such associations—obey and inch). A memory quotient is obtained from a compilation of performance on the seven subtests. This memory quotient is interpreted in a manner analagous to the WAIS IQ, with a MQ of 100 being average for age. The WMS is useful in providing an objective measure of memory performance and in providing information to aid in the differential between organic and functional memory disorders.[37,39]

Sentence Repetition Test (F)

This is a test of the immediate recall of sentence length verbal material. The test consists of 26 tape-recorded sentences of increasing length and complexity. The patient must repeat each sentence immediately after presentation. Norms are available to aid in the interpretation of performance by both children and adults.[36]

Benton Visual Retention Test

See tests of constructional ability.

Memory for Designs

See tests of constructional ability.

CONSTRUCTIONAL ABILITY AND PERCEPTION

Bender Gestalt Test (G)

The test materials consist of nine geometric designs selected by Bender[2] from those introduced by the gestalt school of psychology. The patient is directed to reproduce the stimulus design with paper and pencil. A memory aspect may be introduced after completion of the standard administration by requiring the patient to draw the designs again from memory. The designs are sufficiently simple that perfect reproduction is expected by age 12. Errors in reproduction are often scored in the categories of distortion, rotation, integration, and perseveration. Any errors by an adult which are unexplained by physical or sensory limitations, grossly decreased intellectual ability, or a lack of exposure to graphic tasks in the illiterate are assumed to reflect organic dysfunction, particularly of the right posterior hemisphere.[2,22]

Benton Visual Retention Test (G)

This test consists of a series of simple and complex line drawings which are presented to the patient's view for periods of varying duration (5 to 10 seconds). The patient must then reproduce the design after different delay periods (direct copy, immediate reproduction from memory, and reproduction after a delay of 15 seconds). The test was designed to assess visual perception, visual memory, and visuoconstructive ability. It is relatively brief in administration (5 to 25 minutes depending upon the number of forms administered). An objective scoring system and normative cutoff points for control and brain damaged subjects are provided to aid in the interpretation of results.[3]

WAIS Block Designs Subtest (G)

This subtest of the Wechsler test consists of a series of 10 two colored block designs of increasing complexity. The patient must reproduce the design from a picture stimulus using either four or nine blocks. Both speed and accuracy of reproduction are scored, using a well standardized objective scoring system. The test assesses visual motor reproduction and coordination, and tests the ability to construct abstract designs from parts.[21,38]

WAIS Object Assembly Subtest (G)

The test consists of four picture puzzles of varying complexity and degree of visual cuing. The speed and accuracy of reproduction are scored by means of the standard Wechsler scoring method. The task differs somewhat from that on the Block Designs subtest because of the familiarity of the pictures represented by the puzzle items in contrast to the abstract design nature of the Block Designs tasks.[21,38]

The Grassi Block Substitution Test (B)

The test items consist of a series of block designs of increasing complexity. The test differs from the usual block designs tests in that the patient reproduces stimulus designs constructed by the examiner rather than from printed stimuli.[14]

Embedded Figures Test (F)

The test consists of 16 straight line stimulus figures on half sheets of paper. Figures are traced in an "embedded design" presented in the right half of the same sheet. This is a test primarily of visual perception with less emphasis upon perceptual motor coordination. Norms are available for children and adults.[4]

APHASIA BATTERIES

Halstead-Wepman Aphasia Screening Test (E)

This is a rapidly administered (15 minutes) battery of aphasia, anomia, agnosia, agraphia, dysarthria, and paraphasia. The test is not standardized and its clinical use requires some experience in the interpretation of results of patients with various levels of intelligence, education, and socioeconomic background.[16]

Boston Diagnostic Aphasia Examination (D)

This is a comprehensive examination of aphasia and related cortical disturbance which utilizes a psycholinguistic and multidisciplinary approach. The test was designed to provide both insight into the patient's language functioning and a bridge to relating standard test scores to common aphasic syndromes as recognized by clinical neurologists.[11]

Porch Index of Communicative Ability (C)

The Porch (or PICA) is a comprehensive and highly standardized assessment of language, gestural, and graphic abilities for use with adult aphasics. The test requires a rather lengthy administration time (1.5 hours) and considerable training and experience for the examiner. Scoring criteria are rigid, allowing test-retest and pretreatment and posttreatment comparisons.[23]

Examining for Aphasia (G)

Eisensen's test is another comprehensive battery of tests for the evaluation of language and related disturbance. The test is divided into sections assessing receptive disturbances, including the aphasias and agnosias, and a section evaluating expressive disturbances, including the aphasias and apraxias.[9]

Minnesota Test of Aphasia (G, I)

The Minnesota is a series of 47 subtests of auditory disturbances, speech and language disturbances, visual motor and writing disturbances and disturbances of numerical relations and arithmetic processes. The interpretation of these test results is based upon Schuell's categories of aphasia as defined by the nature and severity of the disturbance. This system, while popular in some sections of the country, is at odds with the classic neuroanatomic categories of aphasia most familiar to neurologists and used in many research centers.[33]

The Token Test (F)

The Token Test is a sensitive test to differentiate between aphasic and nonaphasic populations and to assess the comprehension defect in aphasic patients.[7,20]

AUDITORY PERCEPTION

Seashore Rhythm Test (E, G)

The Rhythm Test is a subtest of the Seashore Measures of Musical Talent and has become a standard component of the Halstead-Reitan Battery. The patient is required to indicate whether a series of 30 pairs of rhythmic beats are the same or different.[28,34]

Wepman Auditory Discrimination Test (I)

The test consists of 40 word pairs equated for length; 30 of the pairs differ in a single phomene, while 10 pairs are identical. The patient must indicate whether the spoken pair is the same or different.[40]

OTHER TESTS OF COGNITIVE DYSFUNCTION

Trail Making Test (E)

This test is a part of the Halstead-Reitan battery which involves two somewhat different tasks. In form A, 25 small circles are randomly printed on a sheet of paper and numbered from 1 to 25. The patient must connect the numbered circles in numerical order as rapidly as possible. In form B, 25 randomly printed circles are numbered from 1 to 13 and lettered from A to L. The patient draws a connecting line, alternating between numbers and letters (i.e., 1-A-2-B-3-C . . .). Form A is generally assumed to be a right hemisphere task, involving primarily perceptual motor speed, while form B is considered a left hemisphere task which requires efficiency in conceptual shifting in addition to perceptual motor speed. This brief (five minute) test is alledged to be sensitive to both diffuse and lateralized brain damage and is often helpful in screening frontal lobe functions.[26,27]

Symbol Digit Modalities Test (I)

This is a briefly administered (five minutes) test involving the conversion of meaningless geometric designs into written and/or spoken number responses. The test is similar in concept to the coding or digit symbol subtests of the Wechsler series. The test is reported to be sensitive to the effects of brain lesions in both children and adults.[35]

Finger Tapping Test (E)

The Finger Tapping Test is a component of the Halstead-Reitan Battery and is also commonly used in various forms in the standard clinical neurologic examination. This technique is well standardized by Reitan among others and requires the patient to tap a mechanical counter with the index finger of each hand. Three trials of 10 seconds each are used for each hand. An averaged score is then obtained for the two hands; these scores are then compared with norms for age and hand dominance. Significant discrepancies between expected norms and actual performance by either hand or discrepancies exceeding 10 percent between hands are considered diagnostic.[28,29]

Proverbs Test (H)

There are many forms of the proverbs test. All are tests of verbal abstract ability and educational knowledge in which the patient either explains the meaning of proverbs or choses the best explanation among a series of choices. The advantages of using this test over the traditional clinical use of proverb interpretation is that these proverbs are graded in difficulty and the responses (both abstract and concrete) are normed. This allows a quantification of performance by the individual patient and a more systematic comparison with expected performance.[12]

Category Test (E)

The Category Test is a significant component of the Halstead-Reitan battery which assesses abstract thinking and problem solving behavior. The patient is required to abstract principles and to learn sorting behavior based upon variables such as size, shape, number, position, brightness, and color.[28,29]

ACHIEVEMENT

Wide Range Achievement Test (G, I)

This is a briefly administered (15 to 20 minutes) test of achievement in the areas of reading (word recognition), spelling to dictation, and written arithmetic. Test items are steeply graded in difficulty, with the test being useable between the grade levels of kindergarten and college. It is useful when a standardized and more objective assessment of deficits in reading, spelling, and calculation ability is needed.[18]

Peabody Individual Achievement Test (A)

This is a well standardized achievement battery with high examinee interest level. The test evaluates performance in the areas of reading recognition, reading comprehension, spelling, arithmetic, and general information. The test is useable through grade 12.9, but because of the nature of its format tends to be more appealing to children than adults.[8]

PERSONALITY

Minnesota Multiphasic Personality Inventory (MMPI) (G)

The MMPI is the most commonly used standardized test of personality. The test consists of 566 statements (e.g., I seldom worry about my health) to which the patient responds true or false as they apply to him. The protocol is then objectively scored, with the resultant profile graphically showing performance in the clinical areas of hypochondriasis, depression, hysteria, psychopathic deviancy, masculinity-femininity of interests, paranoia, psychasthenia (obsessive-compulsive thinking), schizophrenia, hypomania, and social introversion. Validity scales L (lie), F (attempts to "fake bad"), and K (a supressor variable reflecting attempts to "fake good") are also obtained. A number of guidebooks to aid the examiner in interpretation of the significance of individual MMPI configural profiles are available. There are some suggestions that the test may be useful in differentiating organic from functional states and as a lateralizing index for organics.[5,10,17]

Incomplete Sentence Blank (G)

The ISB appears in several forms, all of which consist of a series of sentence stems (e.g., I like ____) which the patient completes. The test is a semiprojective measure of how the patient views himself, his environment, and the people in his environment. Formal administration requires approximately 30 minutes, but may be accomplished in the waiting room with minimal direction and supervision.[31]

REFERENCES

1. Ammons, R., and Ammons, C.: The Quick Test (QT): Provisional Manual. Psychological Test Specialists, Missoula, Mont., 1962.
2. Bender, L.: A Visual Motor Gestalt Test and Its Clinical Use. Research Monograph No. 3, The American Orthopsychiatric Association, New York, 1939.
3. Benton, A.: Benton Revised Visual Retention Test. The Psychological Corporation, New York, 1974.
4. Benton, A., and Spreen, O.: Three-Dimensional Constructional Praxis: A Clinical Test: revised Procedure and Norms. University of Victoria Neuropsychology Laboratory, Victoria, British Columbia, 1966.
5. Black, W.: Unilateral brain lesions and MMPI performance: A preliminary study. Percept. Mot. Skills 40:87, 1975.
6. Burke, H.: Raven's progressive matrices: A review and critical evaluation. J. Genet. Psychol. 93:199, 1958.
7. De Renzi, E., and Vignolo, L.: The token test: A sensitive test to detect receptive disturbances in aphasia. Brain 85:665, 1962.
8. Dunn, L., and Markwardt, F.: Peabody Individual Achievement Test. American Guidance Service, Circle Pines, Minnesota, 1970.
9. Eisensen, J.: Examining for Aphasia. The Psychological Corporation, New York, 1954.
10. Good, P., and Banter, J. The Physician's Guide to the MMPI. University of Minnesota Press, Minneapolis, 1961.
11. Goodglass, H., and Kaplan, E.: The Assessment of Aphasia and Related Disorders. Lea & Febiger, Philadelphia, 1972.
12. Gorham, D.: The Proverbs Test. Psychological Test Specialists, Missoula, Montana, 1956.
13. Graham, F., and Kendall, B.: Memory for designs test: Revised general manual. Percept. Mot. Skills 11:147, 1960.
14. Grassi, J.: The Grassi Block Substitution Test for Measuring Brain Damage. Charles C Thomas, Springfield, Illinois, 1953.
15. Halstead, W.: Brain and Intelligence: A Quantitative Study of the Frontal Lobes. University of Chicago Press, Chicago, 1947.
16. Halstead, W., and Wepman, J.: The Halstead-Wepmann aphasia screening test. J. Speech Hear. Disord. 14:9, 1949.
17. Hathaway, S., and McKinley, J.: Minnesota Multiphasic Personality Inventory. The Psychological Corporation, New York, 1951.
18. Jastak, J., and Jastak, S.: The Wide Range Achievement Test. Guidance Associates, Wilmington, Delaware, 1965.
19. Kent, G.: Series of Emergency Scales: Manual. The Psychological Corporation, New York, 1946.
20. Lesser, R.: Verbal-comprehension in aphasia: An English version of three Italian tests. Cortex 10:247, 1974.
21. Matarazzo, J.: Wechsler's Measurement and Appraisal of Adult Intelligence. Williams & Wilkins, Baltimore, 1972.
22. Pascal, G., and Suttell, B.: The Bender Gestalt Test. Grune & Stratton, New York, 1951.

23. Porch, B.: Porch Index of Communicative Ability. Consulting Psychologists Press, Palo Alto, 1971.
24. Raven, J.: Raven Progressive Matrices. The Psychological Corporation, New York, 1956.
25. Reitan, R.: Investigation of the validity of Halstead's measures of biological intelligence. Arch. Neurol. Psychiatry 48:474, 1955.
26. Reitan, R.: The relation of the trail making test to organic brain damage. J. Consult. Psychol. 19:393, 1955.
27. Reitan, R.: Validity of the trail making test as an indicator of organic brain damage. Percept. Mot. Skills 8:271, 1958.
28. Reitan, R.: The effects of brain lesions on adaptive abilities in human beings (mimeo). Indiana University Medical Center Indianapolis, Indiana, 1959.
29. Reitan, R.: A research program on the psychological effects of brain lesions in human beings, in Ellis, N. (ed.): International Review of Research in Mental Retardation, Vol. 1. Academic Press, New York, 1966, pp. 153-218.
30. Reitan, R., and Davidson, L. (eds.): Clinical Neuropsychology: Current Status and Applications. John Wiley & Sons, New York, 1974.
31. Rotter, J.: Rotter Incomplete Sentence Blank. The Psychological Corporation, New York, 1950.
32. Russell, E., Neuringer, C., and Goldstein, G.: Assessment of brain damage. Wiley-Interscience, New York, 1970.
33. Schuell, H.: Differential Diagnosis of Aphasia with the Minnesota Test. University of Minnesota Press, Minneapolis, 1965.
34. Seashore, C., Lewis, D., and Staetveit, J.: Seashore Measures of Musical Talents. The Psychological Corporation, New York, 1939.
35. Smith, A.: Symbol Digit Modalities Test. Western Psychological Services, Los Angeles, 1973.
36. Spreen, O., and Benton, A.: Sentence Repetition Test: Administration, Scoring, and Preliminary Norms. University of Victoria Neuropsychology Laboratory, Victoria, British Colombia, 1963.
37. Wechsler, D.: A standard memory scale for clinical use. J. Psychol. 19:87, 1945.
38. Wechsler, D.: The Wechsler Adult Intelligence Scale. The Psychological Corporation, New York, 1955.
39. Wechsler, D., and Stone, C.: Wechsler memory scale. The Psychological Corporation, New York, 1973.
40. Wepman, J.: Auditory Discrimination Test: 1973 Revision. Western Psychological Services, Los Angeles, 1973.

APPENDIX 2

Composite Mental Status Examination

Date_____

Patient Name _____Age_____Diagnosis_____

Occupation_____Education_____

(Starred items are essential and should be used with all patients.)

*I.   Level of Consciousness

    *A. Rate: Alert_____ Lethargic_____ Stupor_____ Coma_____

    *B. Describe Patient's Condition:

*II.   Behavioral Observations

    *A. History:

    *B. Physical Appearance:

    *C. Emotional Status:

    D. Frontal Lobe Test Results:

*III. Attention

    *A. Observation:

    *B. Digit Repetition:

Item	Check if Correct
1. 3-7	_____
2. 2-4-9	_____
3. 8-5-2-1	_____
4. 2-9-6-8-3	_____
5. 5-7-1-9-4-6	_____
6. 8-1-5-9-3-6-2	_____
7. 3-9-8-2-5-1-4-7	_____
8. 7-2-8-5-4-6-7-3-9	_____

    C. Vigilence:

      L T P E A O A I C T D A L A A

      A N I A B F S A M R Z E O A D

      P A K L A U C J T O E A B A A

      Z Y F M U S A H E V A A R A T

    1. Errors of Omission: _____

    2. Errors of Commission: _____

    D. Unilateral Inattention and Neglect:

*IV. Language

    *A. Handedness:

      *1. Self   _____

      *2. Family _____

    *B. Spontaneous Speech:

      Describe including types of errors:

    *C. Comprehension:

      *1. Patient's response to pointing commands:

*2. Patient's response to yes-no questions:

*D. Repetition:

Item	Check if Correct
1. Ball	_____
2. Help	_____
3. Airplane	_____
4. Hospital	_____
5. Mississippi River	_____
6. The little boy went home	_____
7. We all went over there together	_____
8. Let's go downtown for ice cream	_____
9. The short fat boy dropped the china vase	_____
10. Each fight readied the boxer for the championship bout	_____

*E. Naming and Word Finding:

Item	Check if Correct
1. Colors	
a. Red	_____
b. Blue	_____
c. Yellow	_____
d. Pink	_____
e. Purple	_____
2. Body Parts	
f. Eye	_____
g. Leg	_____
h. Teeth	_____
i. Thumb	_____
j. Knuckles	_____
3. Clothing & Room Objects	
k. Door	_____
l. Watch	_____
m. Shoe	_____
n. Shirt	_____
o. Ceiling	_____
4. Parts of Objects	
p. Watch Stem (Winder)	_____
q. Coat Lapel	_____

      r. Watch Crystal   _____

      s. Sole of Shoe   _____

      t. Buckle of Belt   _____

F. Reading:

Describe level of adequacy (words, sentences, paragraphs) and note types of errors:

G. Writing:

Describe level of adequacy and note types of errors:

H. Spelling:

Describe performance and note errors:

*V.   Memory

   *A. Immediate Recall (Short Term Memory):

      Refer to Digit Repetition in Section III

   *B. Orientation:

                                   Check if Correct

      *1. Person

          a. Name   _____

          b. Age   _____

          c. Birthdate   _____

      *2. Place

          a. Location   _____

          b. Home Address   _____

          c. City Location   _____

      *3. Time

          a. Date   _____

          b. Day of the Week   _____

          c. Time of Day   _____

          d. Season of the Year _____

          e. Duration of Time   _____

*C. Remote Memory:

Check if Correct
or Adequate

  *1. Personal Information
     a. Where were you born?   _____
     b. School Information   _____
     c. Vocational History   _____
     d. Family Information   _____

  *2. Historical Facts
     a. Four Presidents   _____
     b. Last War   _____

*D. New Learning Ability:

  1. Four Unrelated
     Words   5 minutes   10 minutes   30 minutes

	5 minutes	10 minutes	30 minutes
a. Brown	_____	_____	_____
b. Honesty	_____	_____	_____
c. Tulip	_____	_____	_____
d. Eyedropper	_____	_____	_____

Describe type of cues used if necessary:

  2. Verbal Story for Immediate Recall:

    William Stern / a 63 year old / state representative / from Walton County / Utah / was planning his reelection campaign / when he began experiencing chest pain./ He entered Logan Memorial Hospital / for three days of medical tests./ A harmless virus was diagnosed / and he, his wife / Sandra, / and their two sons / Rick and Tommy / hit the campaign trail again./

     a. Number of correct memories: _____
     b. Describe confabulation if present:

  3. Visual Memory (Hidden Objects):

     a. Number of hidden objects found: _____
     b. Number of hidden objects named if not
        found: _____

4. Visual Memory (Visual Design Reproduction):

Item	Score
a. Design 1	_____
b. Design 2	_____
c. Design 3	_____
d. Design 4	_____

Total Score _____

5. Paired Associate Learning:

Presentation Lists

1	2
a. Weather—Bag	a. House—Income
b. High—Low	b. Weather—Bag
c. House—Income	c. Book—Page
d. Book—Page	d. High—Low

Recall Lists

1		2	
a. House	_____	a. High	_____
b. High	_____	b. House	_____
c. Weather	_____	c. Book	_____
d. Book	_____	d. Weather	_____

1. Number of easy paired associates recalled:

_____

2. Number of difficult paired associates recalled:

_____

*VI. Constructional Ability

*A. Reproduction Drawings:

Item	Score
1. Horizontal Diamond	_____
2. Two Dimensional Cross	_____
3. Three Dimensional Cube	_____
4. Three Dimensional Pipe	_____

Total Score: _____

*B. Drawings to Command:

Item	Score
1. Clock	_____
2. Daisy in Flower Pot	_____
3. House in Perspective	_____

Total Score: _____

C. Block Designs:

Item	Score
1. Design 1	_____
2. Design 2	_____
3. Design 3	_____
4. Design 4	_____

Total Score: _____

Describe types of errors:

*VII. Higher Cognitive Functions

A. Fund of Information:

Item	Check if Correct
1. How many weeks are in the year?	_____
2. Why do people have lungs?	_____
3. Name four presidents since 1940.	_____
4. Where is Luxembourg?	_____
5. How far is it from New York to Los Angeles?	_____
6. Why are light colored clothes cooler in the summer than dark colored clothes?	_____
7. What is the capitol of Spain?	_____
8. What causes rust?	_____
9. Who wrote the Odyssey?	_____
10. What is the Acropolis?	_____

Total Score: _____

*B. Proverb Interpretation:

Item	Score
1. Rome wasn't built in a day.	_____

2. A drowning man will clutch at a straw. _____

3. A golden hammer breaks an iron door. _____

4. The hot coal burns, the cold one blackens. _____

Total Score: _____

Total Concrete Responses: _____

*C. Similarities:

Item	Score
1. Turnip . . . . . . Califlower	_____
2. Desk . . . . Bookcase	_____
3. Poem . . . . Novel	_____
4. Horse . . . . Apple	_____

Total Score: _____

Total Concrete Responses: _____

*D. Calculations:

Describe the patient's adequacy in performance and types of errors made on the following types of calculations:

1. Verbal Rote Examples

    a. Addition   (3 + 3)
    b. Subtraction   (9 − 2)
    c. Multiplication   (5 × 5)
    d. Division   (56 ÷ 8)

2. Verbal Complex Examples

    a. Addition   (14 + 17)
    b. Subtraction   (43 − 38)
    c. Multiplication   (21 × 5)
    d. Division   (128 ÷ 8)

*3. Written Complex Examples

    a. Addition   (108 + 79)
    b. Subtraction   (605 − 86)
    c. Multiplication   (108 × 36)
    d. Division   (348 ÷ 6)

E. Conceptual Series Completion:

Item	Check if Correct
1. 1 4 7 10 __ __	_____
2. AZ BY CX D __	_____
3. tote to snow on spun up stab __ __	_____
4. elephant 87654321 plan 5732 lap	_____

__ __ __

Total Score: _____

VIII. Related Cortical Functions

A. Ideomotor Apraxia:

Describe the adequacy of the patient's performance in carrying out motor acts to command using buccofacial, limb, and whole body commands. Indicate if imitation or use of the real object was necessary to facilitate performance.

B. Ideational Apraxia:

Describe the adequacy of the patient's performance on the following complex motor tasks:

1. Letter—Envelope—Stamp
2. Candle—Holder—Match
3. Toothpaste—Brush

C. Right—Left Disorientation:

Item	Check if Correct
1. Identification on Self	
a. Show me your right foot.	_____
b. Show me your left hand.	_____
2. Crossed Commands on Self	
a. With your right hand touch your left shoulder	_____
b. With your left hand touch your right ear	_____
3. Identification on Examiner	
a. Point to my left knee	_____
b. Point to my right elbow	_____

4. Crossed Commands on Examiner

   a. With your right hand point to
      my left eye   _____

   b. With your left hand point to
      my left foot   _____

Describe nature and degree of errors made:

D. Finger Agnosia:

Describe adequacy of the patient's performance in identifying named fingers on the examiner's hand and in verbally naming fingers on self:

E. Gerstmann Syndrome:

Describe the nature and degree of impairment in the following areas if present in the patient:

1. Finger Agnosia:

2. Right-Left Disorientation:

3. Dysgraphia:

4. Dyscalculia:

F. Visual Agnosia:

Describe any deficits in visual identification of objects, naming of objects whose use can be demonstrated, color naming, and facial recognition:

G. Geographic Orientation:

    1. Describe evidence of disorientation obtained from history:

    2. Map Localization:

    Describe patient's ability to localize well known cities on a map:

    3. Orientation of Self in Hospital:

    Describe the patient's ability to orient himself within the hospital environment:

SUMMARY OF FINDINGS

1. Describe major areas of impairment:

2. Tentative neurobehavioral diagnosis:

3. Tentative localization:

4. Tentative clinical diagnosis:

5. Proposed management plans:

Index

175

Constructional apraxia, 86
Constructional impairment, 86
  clinical implications of, 102-105
  tests for, 86
Constructional praxis, 85
Contralateral inattention, 22
Corpus callosum, lesion of
  anterior, 57
  alexia in, 55
Cortex
  abstract functions and 115
  atrophy of, psychiatric symptomology and, 3
  disease of, bilateral, constructional impairment with, 103
  dysfunction of, in acute confusional state, 31
  extensive bilateral damage to and diffuse brain dysfunction, 21
  functions of, related, 119-132
  lesion of, pure dysarthria in, 54
  mantle of, diffuse damage to, 12
  multiple infarcts of, and frontal lobe syndrome, 34
  stimulation of, and attention, 20

DEAFNESS, pure word, 54
Dejà vu in temporal lobe epilepsy, 34
Delirium, toxic, 30
Dementia
  Alzheimer's, memory deficit in, 79
  atrophic, remote memory loss in, 81
  organic, advanced, psychotic language in, 57-59
  multiple infarct, constructional impairment with, 103
  senile, 135-136
    presenile and, memory loss in, 63
    short term memory and, 78
Denial
  neglect and, 35-37
  organic, 18
Depersonalization in temporal lobe epilepsy, 34
Depression
  vs. apathy, 34-35
  in Broca's aphasia, 50
  inattention and, 22
  memory loss in, 63-64
  nonreactive and reactive, 3
Diffuse brain dysfunction and inattention, 21
Digit recall, 77-78
Digit repetition test for attentiveness, 18-19
Disconnection syndrome(s), 51
Disinterest in family or work, organic brain disease and, 4

Disorientation, right-left, 125-126
Dissociative state, memory disturbance in, 82
Distractability, 17-18
Dominant hemisphere lesions, 134
Double simultaneous stimulation test for inattention and neglect, 19-20
Drawings to command test, 89-95
Drug
  intoxication
    diffuse brain dysfunction, and 21
    reticular and cortical function and, 11
  reaction to, in acute confusional state, 30
Dysarthria, 39
  pure, 54-55
Dyscalculia, 116
Dysfluency, 55
Dyslexia, 40
Dyspraxia, sympathetic, 122
Dysprosody, 39-40

ECHOLALIA in transcortical aphasia, 53
Elderly patients
  acute confusional state and, 31
  psychotic language in, 57-59
Embedded Figures Test, 155-156
Emotional change in Broca's aphasia, 50
Emotional status in behavior evaluation, 26-27
Encephalitis, 21
  herpes simplex, organic amnesia in, 79
Encephalopathy
  anoxic, visual agnosia in, 128
  postinfectious, in frontal lobe syndrome, 34
  toxic, 30
  Wernicke's, and Korsakoff's syndrome, 79
Epilepsy, temporal lobe, 34
Euphoria in frontal lobe syndrome, 32
Examination, Composite Mental Status, 163-173
Examining for aphasia, 156
Exogenous reaction, acute, 30
Expressive aphasics, 48
Extinction, test for, 19-20

FAMILY counseling, 149
Finger agnosia, 126-127
Finger Tapping Test, 158
Fist-palm-side test, 28
Fist-ring test, 28
Frontal lobe
  bilateral lesions of
    apathy in, 34
    inattention and, 21
  deep, tumor of, 12
  syndrome, 32-34

177

Frustration in Broca's aphasia, 50
Fugue state, 82
Fund of information test, 108-109

GANSER syndrome, 82
Geographic orientation, 129-131
Gerstmann syndrome, 57, 127-128
  dyscalculia in, 116
Global aphasia, 49
Grasp reflex, 12
Grassi Block Substitution Test, 155
Gross explicit denial, 36

HALLUCINATIONS
  auditory, and functional confusional
    state, 31
  visual
    auditory or, in temporal lobe epilepsy, 34
    organic confusional state and, 31
Halstead-Reitan Battery, 152
Halstead-Wepman Aphasia Screening Test,
  156
Handedness, 40-41
Head trauma, 21
  acute, amnesia after, 79-80
  in frontal lobe syndrome, 33
Heart failure, confusion in, 31
Hemiplegia, global aphasia and, 49
Hemorrhage of reticular formation, 9
Hepatic failure, confusion in, 31
Heredity and cerebral dominance for
  language, 41
Herniation, hippocampal and uncal, leth-
  argy and, 11
Higher cognitive functions, 107-118
Hippocampus
  bilateral infarction of, organic amnesia
    and, 79
  herniation of, and lethargy, 11
Huntington's chorea in frontal lobe syn-
  drome, 33
Hydrocephalus
  communicating, in frontal lobe syndrome,
    33
  psychiatric symptomology and, 3
Hypoglycemia and cortical mantle, 12
Hyposexuality, global, in temporal lobe epi-
  lepsy, 34
Hypothalamus, anterior, lesions of, and
  akinetic mutism, 12
Hysteric coma-like state, 14
Hysterical neurosis, 82

ICTAL phenomena, 34
Ideational apraxia, 124-125
Ideomotor apraxia, 119-124
Inattention, 17-18
  contralateral, 22
  memory testing and, 81

short term memory and, 78
test for, 19-20
unilateral, 18
  in midbrain lesions, 21
Incomplete Sentence Blank, 159-160
Infarct(s)
  cortical, 21
    multiple, and frontal lobe syndrome, 34
  mental status examination and, 2
  of reticular formation, 9
Infection, systemic, and diffuse brain dysfunction, 21
Insight therapy, 149
Intelligence tests, 152-153
Interictal phenomena, 34
Intoxication
  drug, and diffuse brain dysfunction, 21
  reticular and cortical function and, 11
Intracranial pressure, increased, in acute
  confusional state, 31
Irritability in frontal lobe syndrome, 32
Isolation syndrome, 53

JARGON aphasia, 42
  differentiation from, 57-59

KENT Series of Emergency Scales, 152
Korsakoff's syndrome
  memory deficit in, 79
  remote memory in, 81

LANGUAGE, 39-61
  disorders, nonorganic, 59-60
  evaluation of, 40-47
  psychotic, 57-59
  speech and, evaluation of, 144-145
Left hand
  cerebral dominance in, 47
  pathways for praxis in, 122-123
  pure agraphia with, 57
Left parietal lobe patients, constructional
  impairment in, 102-103
Lesion
  anterior borderzone, 53
  of anterior corpus callosum, 57
  anterior hypothalamic, 12
  of anterior speech area, 49
  of arcurate fasciculus, 50
  of ascending activating system, 21
  of basal ganglia, 54
  bilateral
    of frontal lobes, 21
    of limbic system, 21
    of orbital frontal cortex, 12
  brain, neuropsychologic evaluation and,
    140-142
  of bulbar neurons, 54
  of cingulate gyri, 12
  of corpus callosum, 55

178

PANENCEPHALITIS, subacute sclerosing, 116
Paramnesia in denial, 35
Paranoia in temporal lobe epilepsy, 34
Paraphasias, 41, 42
Paresis in frontal lobe syndrome, 33
Parietal lobes
  in constructional ability, 102
  lesion(s)
    focal dominant, 117
    in Wernicke's aphasia, 50
Parietotemporal area, lesions of, 52
Parkinsonism, pure dysarthria in, 54
Peabody Individual Achievement Test, 159
Perception, tests for, 154-156
Perisylvian cortex, parietal, repetition and, 53
Perseveration, 21-22
Persistent vegetative state, 12
Personality, tests of, 159-160
Phonemic paraphasia, 42
Physical appearance in behavior evaluation, 25-26
Physical complaints without organic etiology, organic brain disease and, 4
Pick's dementia, 33
  remote memory loss in, 81
Pituitary adenomas in frontal lobe syndrome, 33
Pons, lesions of, and inattention, 21
Pontine lesion, 12
  pure dysarthria in, 54
Porch Index of Communicative Ability, 156
Postneurosurgical evaluation, 140
Postsurgical states and diffuse brain dysfunction, 21
Praxis, pathways for
  in left hand, 122-123
  in right hand, 122
Preneurosurgical evaluation, 140
Presenile dementia, memory loss in, 63
Primitive reflexes, 12
Progressive Matrices Test, 152-153
Prosopagnosia, 129
Proverb interpretation test, 109-111
Proverbs Test, 158
Pseudobulbar palsy, pure dysarthria in, 54
Pseudodementia, 35
  memory disturbance in, 82
Psychiatric disease, organic and, differentiation of, 3-4
Psychiatric patients, mental status examination and, 3
Psychiatry, 146-149
  referral for evaluation, 146-148
  treatment with, 148-149
Psychogenic unresponsiveness, 14
Psychologic tests, standard, 151-161
Psychologists as expert witnesses, 140-141

Psychosis
  severe functional, psychotic language in, 57-59
  Wernicke's aphasia and, 50
Psychotic language, 57-59
Pulmonary failure, confusion in, 31
Pure dysarthria, 54-55
Pure word deafness, 54

QUICK Test, 153

RANDOM letter test for vigilance, 19
Reading ability, 45-46
Recall, immediate, 77-78
  evaluation of, 66
Receptive aphasics, 48
Reciprocal coordination test, 28-30
Reduplication
  of body parts, in denial, 35
  of place, in denial, 35
Referral
  to neuropsychologist, 140-141
  for psychiatric evaluation, 146-148
  to speech pathologist, 143-144
Reflex (es)
  increased, in legs, 12
  primitive, 12
Rehabilitation, neurobehavioral sequelae and, 2
Related cortical functions, 119-132
Religious interest, increased, in temporal lobe epilepsy, 34
Repetition
  and perisylvian cortex, 53
  of spoken language, 44-45
Reproduction drawings tests, 87-89
Reticular activating system, brain stem, 20
Reticular neurons, specialized, 9
Right hand
  cerebral dominance in, 47
  pathways for praxis in, 122
Right hemisphere, lesions of
  apathy in, 34
  inattention and, 22
Right-left disorientation, 125-126
Right parietal lobe patients, constructional impairment in, 102-103

SCHIZOPHRENIA
  impaired abstracting ability and, 117
  psychotic language in, 57-59
Schizophreniform psychosis in temporal lobe epilepsy, 34
Seashore Rhythm Test, 157
Semantic paraphasia, 42
Semicoma, 8
Senile dementia, 135-136
  constructional impairment with, 103